W9-AWP-092

New Technology
in Nursing Staff Development

Choosing, Justifying, and Implementing
Nontraditional Teaching Methods

Reviewed by
Diane Billings, EdD, RN, FAAN

HCPro

Diane Billings, EdD, RN, FAAN, Reviewer
Cynthia Hollingsworth, MS, BS, AAS, Author
Kathie Lasater, EdD, RN, Author
Jesika Gavilanes, MA, Author
Dorothea Devanna, MS, ACNS-BC, Author
Emily Sheahan, Group Publisher
Rebecca Hendren, Senior Managing Editor
Lindsey Cardarelli, Associate Editor

Dennis Ludvino, Layout Artist
Mike Mirabello, Senior Graphic Artist
Leah Tracosas, Copyeditor
Patrick Campagnone, Cover Designer
Erika Bryan, Proofreader
Darren Kelly, Books Production Supervisor
Susan Darbyshire, Art Director
Jean St. Pierre, Director of Operations

Advice given is general. Readers should consult professional counsel for specific legal, ethical, or clinical questions. Arrangements can be made for quantity discounts. For more information, contact:

HCPro, Inc.
P.O. Box 1168
Marblehead, MA 01945
Telephone: 800/650-6787 or 781/639-1872
Fax: 781/639-2982
E-mail: *customerservice@hcpro.com*

Visit HCPro at its World Wide Web sites:
www.hcpro.com and *www.hcmarketplace.com*

Table of contents

Chapter 4: Blended learning 71

List of figures

Diane Billings, EdD, RN, FAAN

Diane Billings, EdD, RN, FAAN, is chancellor's professor emeritus of nursing at Indiana University School of Nursing in Indianapolis. As a consultant and freelance instructional designer, she works with educator groups to integrate best practices in teaching and learning in online courses.

Billings is the author of three award-winning nursing textbooks and has published articles in nursing and higher education journals in the area of using information technology to support teaching and learning. She is the recipient of national awards for her teaching and innovative use of technology. She serves on the editorial boards of five nursing journals. Her current research focuses on benchmarking best practices in teaching and learning.

About the authors

Cynthia Hollingsworth, MS, BS, AAS

Cynthia Hollingsworth, MS, BS, AAS, is the coordinator of instructional design and an adjunct assistant faculty at the Indiana University School of Nursing in Indianapolis. She supports nursing faculty and frequently consults with schools and organizations as they move to Web-based learning. Her emphasis is on effective design, active learning strategies, instructional technologies, and principles of adult learning. She has presented at multiple national conferences on these topics including the National Nursing Staff Development Organization and Learning Resources Centers conferences and the National Academy of Infusion Therapy's annual meeting.

Hollingsworth serves on the editorial board for the International Nursing Association for Clinical Simulation and Learning (INACSL). Cynthia contributed two chapters to *Conversations in E-learning*, an AJN Book of the Year for Nursing Education and Continuing Education, published by Pohl Publishing in 2002. She is a member of INACSL, the International Webmasters Association, and a senior member in the Society for Technical Communication.

Kathie Lasater, EdD, RN

Kathie Lasater, EdD, RN, is an assistant professor at the Oregon Health and Science University (OHSU) School of Nursing in Portland and recently served as Interim Statewide Director of Simulation Learning for the university's five campuses. As one of the first nurse researchers exploring mannequin-based simulation and its impact on students' development of clinical judgment, Lasater helped to shape the OHSU simulation program's focus on clinical judgment (or "thinking like a nurse").

For the past five years, Lasater has been involved in curriculum development and research and evaluation of the Oregon Consortium for Nursing Education (OCNE), an innovative model of nursing education that brings together baccalaureate and associate degree programs as well as service institutions to revolutionize nursing education for the 21st century.

In 2007, Lasater received the Outstanding Baccalaureate Faculty Award for Excellence in Teaching. In 2008, she was inducted as a fellow in the Academy of Nursing Education.

Jesika Gavilanes, MA

Jesika Gavilanes, MA, is the operations manager of the Oregon Health and Science University (OHSU) Simulation and Clinical Learning Center. Gavilanes has been integral in the design and development of the center's policies, procedures, and infrastructure since its opening in 2002. She provides ongoing technical and faculty support for simulation at the center, in the OHSU hospital, and throughout the state of Oregon.

Gavilanes has presented posters and given presentations at international simulation conferences and has received several awards for outstanding service excellence at OHSU. Most recently, she has developed and implemented a SimTech Academy curriculum for the Oregon Simulation Alliance to train simulation technicians across the state. She has also been a senior consultant with SimHealth Consultants for the past two years.

Dorothea Devanna, MS, ACNS-BC

Dorothea Devanna, MS, ACNS-BC, is a medical-surgical clinical nurse specialist at Mount Auburn Hospital in Cambridge, MA. She is responsible for nursing orientation, continuing education, competency assessment, and staff education within the organization.

Devanna has worked as a staff nurse, nursing supervisor, case manager, and a clinical nurse specialist during her career. She has presented at national conventions on organizational changes she has helped implement at Mount Auburn.

How to use the files on the CD-ROM

The following file names correspond with figures listed in the book *New Technology in Nursing Staff Development: Choosing, Justifying, and Implementing Nontraditional Teaching Methods.*

Fig1-1.rtf	Figure 1.1: Sample letter for use of copyrighted material
Fig1-2.rtf	Figure 1.2: VHS vs. DVD: Advantages and disadvantages
Fig1-3.rtf	Figure 1.3: Request form to preview educational videos
Fig1-4.rtf	Figure 1.4: PowerPoint samples
Fig1-5.rtf	Figure 1.5: Waiver for use of video likeness during a presentation
Fig1-6.rtf	Figure 1.6: Waiver for use of video likeness (for a minor)
Fig1-7.rtf	Figure 1.7: Waiver for use of video likeness (for an adolescent)
Fig1-8.rtf	Figure 1.8: Permission to use copyrighted material (by a videographer)
Fig1-9.rtf	Figure 1.9: Copyright assignment (by a staff or student as a "work-for-hire")
Fig3-1.rtf	Figure 3.1: The STAIR method
Fig4-1.rtf	Figure 4.1: Teaching methods for various learning styles
Fig4-2.rtf	Figure 4.2: Barriers in blended learning
Fig4-3.rtf	Figure 4.3: Blended learning and the different generations
Fig4-4.rtf	Figure 4.4: Basic dysrhythmia interpretation
Fig4-5.rtf	Figure 4.5: Phases of communication
Fig5-1.pdf	Figure 5.1: Logistics check-off list
Fig5-2.pdf	Figure 5.2: An integrative model of clinical judgment
Fig5-3.pdf	Figure 5.3: Sample scenario template
Fig5-4.rtf	Figure 5.4: Evidence-based dimensions of clinical judgment
Fig5-5.rtf	Figure 5.5: Sample debriefing questions by dimension to foster clinical judgment
Fig5-6.pdf	Figure 5.6: Lasater clinical judgment rubric

The following file name is a bonus example found only on the CD-ROM.

Color_Wheel.rtf	Sample color wheel

To adapt any of the files to your own facility, simply follow the instructions below to open the CD.

If you have trouble reading the forms, click on View, and then Normal. To adapt the forms, save them first to your own hard drive or disk (by clicking File, then Save as, and changing the system to your own). Then change the information to fit your facility, and add or delete any items that you wish to change.

Installation instructions

This product was designed for the Windows operating system and includes Word files that will run under Windows 95/98 or greater. The CD will work on all PCs and most Macintosh systems. To run the files on the CD/ROM, take the following steps:

1. Insert the CD into your CD/ROM drive.

2. Double-click on the My Computer icon, next double-click on the CD drive icon.

3. Double-click on the files you wish to open.

4. Adapt the files by moving the cursor over the areas you wish to change, highlighting them, and typing in the new information using Microsoft Word.

5. To save a file to your facility's system, click on File and then click on Save As. Select the location where you wish to save the file and then click on Save.

6. To print a document, click on File and then click on Print.

                   New Technology in Nursing Staff Development

Introduction

Did you ever have the nightmare in which you stand up to teach and realize you still have on your pajamas? Some staff educators have that same sensation when they stand before a classroom of learners and realize that these learners believe that:

- Educators have always written on whiteboards with markers or used overhead projectors rather than chalkboards

- Responses to communication should occur instantaneously (or at least no more than an hour or two after being received)

- Content should be accessible any time, not just during the orientation session

- Resources and lessons should be available through a variety of channels—computer, handouts, audio, and video—not just in the classroom

- Schedules shouldn't have to be rearranged in order to complete an assigned group project

These beliefs can be quite daunting for an educator who was trained and is experienced in traditional classroom instruction. But have no fear! In this book, we'll discuss training as it relates to mainstream and emerging educational technologies. We'll take time to explain tools in ways that make them understandable to those who may have only a passing knowledge or hearsay understanding of them. We will share strategies that educators can adopt and use to implement tools effectively. And we will share the positives and negatives of educational technologies in terms of educator investments of time and money.

The best, "coolest," and most expensive technology is worthless if it is not implemented using sound educational practices and techniques that will help learners master the learning objectives. Therefore, the purpose of this book is to present instructional technologies in such a way that you will understand the tools and how they can be paired with instructional strategies to meet those educational goals.

Instructional technologies can sound daunting to those who may have some reservations about technology. Instead, think of them as tools that teachers use to help learners. Technologies don't have to be high tech. In fact, some of the best teaching tools are decidedly low tech. Instructional technology should be like signage along an interstate—if you don't need it to reach your goal, you never notice it is there; however, if you need extra assistance in reaching your goal, then the technology needs to be easily understood whether you're an expert or a novice. It needs to help you reach your goal with the minimum amount of interference and bother.

Classroom technology has evolved from simple black-painted walls written on with chalk in the early 1800s to the whiteboards and dry erase markers of many of today's classrooms. The ubiquitous overhead projector that made its appearance in most classrooms in the 1960s and continues to be a staple in education today began as the "magic lantern" as long ago as 1874. The first teachers presented with an overhead project or might have protested that they didn't have time to learn to use it; the students were learning just fine with information presented on the chalkboard. Yet, over time, it became difficult to find any educator who has not written on an acetate sheet with a wipe-off marker pen and displayed the information on a wall or screen by an overhead projector.

Each chapter in this book will present one technology or family of technologies and discuss the teaching and learning strategies that you can use to facilitate learners' achievement of the learning goals and objectives. We will share advantages and disadvantages of those tools and strategies. The goal of the book is not your mastery of all of the content but rather to be a grand educational smorgasbord to which you can return time and time again, sampling old favorites, trying new items to see whether they fit your palate, and mixing and matching to blend the old and new, the tried and the unknown.

Audio/visual

After reading this chapter, the participant will be able to:

- Identify advantages of audio/visual technologies

- List roadblocks that may hinder the use of audio/visual media

Many of us may recall sitting in lectures, orientations, or inservices watching movies, each of which always seemed to be identifiable by the same series theme song that would then play repeatedly in our heads. Fortunately, education has changed ... or has it? Much education still uses primarily listen-and-watch-to-learn strategies, even though the specific technologies employed have changed time and time again. This chapter will take you on a bird's-eye view of audio/visual (A/V) technologies from videos to podcasts (and vodcasts). While entire texts have been written to cover these topics, our goal is to introduce each technology to you and to demonstrate some of the advantages and disadvantages of each.

Commercial videos

In the 1950s and 1960s, those movies mentioned earlier in this chapter were usually reel-to-reel filmstrips that clicked as the sprockets drew the strip forward. Occasionally, a film would "jump track," leaving a jumbled pile of film on the floor next to the projector. The sound level was difficult to control; learners in the far corners of the room couldn't hear, and those sitting next to the projector in the back of the classroom dealt with audio levels that were too high. And when the movie finally ended, the filmstrip's end would flap and flap until the educator made it to the back of the room to shut off the projector.

From a teacher's standpoint, one disadvantage to this instructional technology was in starting and stopping the film at strategic points so that discussion could occur at those "teachable moments." This task had to be coordinated carefully: sometimes someone seated near the projector could handle the task while the educator stayed at the front of the room. Other times, the instructor had to manage both the technology and the teaching, moving from the back to the front of the classroom in order to run the projector and to teach. Thus, many educators found it easier to simply let the film play through from beginning to end and then conduct the discussion, which missed those teachable moments.

Enter the 1980s. Educators felt that they had achieved great technological strides when reel-to-reel filmstrips and projectors were upgraded to VCR players and VHS tapes. However, similar issues seemed to prevail: Effective audio levels were difficult to set and maintain, and the tape still, occasionally, malfunctioned, leaving a tape-spaghetti mess, generally in the player so that it had to be pulled out while you hoped that the internal mechanism wasn't being destroyed in the process.

Despite all of this, VHS tapes and VCRs were technological progress. Contained tapes were easier to load into the player, some classrooms included VCRs as standard teaching technologies, and occasionally educators were fortunate enough to have a remote control with which tapes easily could be stopped, started, paused, and rewound. These features allowed more effective educational strategies to be employed, such as strategically pausing the video to lead a discussion, explain concepts, and gauge learner understanding before restarting the tape. Many classrooms continue to use VHS tapes.

In the mid-1990s, DVDs entered mainstream education, usually supplementing rather than replacing existing VHS libraries. The clarity of the projection was enhanced as DVD and the projectors themselves had better video quality.

For face-to-face learning, these audio/video technologies had advantages. They:

- Were portable

New Technology in Nursing Staff Development

- Provided visual and aural enhancement for lessons

- Were easy to use

- Were developed using professional actors and settings for realistic quality

A major disadvantage was replacement costs, both of the media and of the players. A/V media used to teach clinical skills, which are often series or libraries rather than individual tapes, can be quite costly. As video media ages, VHS tapes begin to break down, and without special care, dust, scratches, and body oils on DVD surfaces cause players to skip, blur, or stop playing. In addition, the contents themselves age. Techniques become outdated; social cues such as language, hair, and dress styles do not stay current; and equipment and tools become a generation or more old.

Another disadvantage is that educators seldom find "just the right" media that includes the range of skill, technique, and content needed to assist learners in meeting learning objectives. Sometimes a particular media has some components that are less desirable and other components that are exactly on-target. Or, as media publishers upgrade A/V selections, some components are deleted and new ones added. Schools and healthcare facilities must weigh whether it is more effective to continue using media that is no longer quite as effective as it once was or to expend funds to replace costly media. Educators are left with the quandary of "Do we throw away something that has perfectly good portions just so we can upgrade and get the new stuff, or do we buy media that has mostly what is needed and do without the rest?"

As distributed education began to gain footholds in the 90s, additional issues surrounding the use of commercially published audio and video arose. Educators wished to use the same educational strategies—video media—to reach learners at a distance as they use in face-to-face classrooms. Learners were changing as well. They wanted access to media at times convenient for their learning rather than solely in face-to-face classroom educational sessions. This trend in education continues today.

To provide additional access for learners and educators alike, institutions want to install copies of media on their own servers, create backup copies, and allow media to be accessed from multiple classrooms and offices across an institution. Unfortunately, there are roadblocks:

- Some institutions do not possess the technology to digitize A/V media.

- Publishers are reluctant to grant permission for commercially created media to be replicated, stored, and served via networks rather than delivered from a single media to a single learner or contained classroom of learners.

- When permission is granted, it often is accompanied by restrictions on how long it can be stored on the server, the number of students who are allowed to access it either in total or at a given time, and the duration of the period when any given group of learners have access. Permissions are often granted only with the payment of use fees and include stipulations regarding the need to re-request permission at specified times.

The Copyright Advisory Office of Columbia University Libraries/Information Services Web site (*www.copyright.columbia.edu/model-permissions-letters*) provides guidelines for forming a request letter in order to seek permission to use copyrighted materials. In addition to recommending that requests be mailed (although e-mail requests are legal) with a valid signature and accompanied by a self-addressed, stamped return envelope, the Copyright Advisory Office 2008 also states these important criteria:

> *Describe precisely the proposed use of the copyrighted material. If necessary or appropriate, attach a copy of the quotations, diagrams, pictures, and other materials. If the proposed use is extensive, such as the general use of an archival or manuscript collection, describe it in broad yet reasonably specific terms. Your objectives are to eliminate any ambiguities and to be sure the permission encompasses the full scope of your needs.*

Figure 1.1 is a sample letter for requesting the use of copyrighted material. It is used with permission from the Copyright Advisory Office. Figure 1.1 shows an example of how you might use the sample to request permission to digitize a DVD so that it can be made accessible to your distance learners. Notice that it is not necessary to follow the form exactly but rather to provide specific details pertinent to your unique situation and to include sufficient details that an informed consent can be provided.

 New Technology in Nursing Staff Development

FIGURE
1.1

Sample letter for use of copyrighted material

June 20, 2008

Cynthia D. Hollingsworth
Coordinator of Instructional Design
Adjunct Assistant Faculty
Indiana University School of Nursing
1111 Middle Drive, NU 452B
Indianapolis, IN 46202

ABC Publishing, Inc.
123 E. Main Street
New York, NY 00000

Re: Basic Perioperative Techniques

Dear Permissions Editor:

I am on the faculty of Indiana University School of Nursing where I teach in the Environments for Health department. I teach basic perioperative nursing to first-semester sophomore nursing students. I currently show "Demonstrating Opening a Sterile Package" portion of the *Basic Perioperative Techniques* DVD in my face-to-face class. I believe that you hold the copyright to this work and that it would have important educational value for my students. Beginning in fall 2008, we will be pilot-test offering this course to 20 students via our Web-based course management system. I would like your permission to have our information services staff digitize the 8-minute segment of this DVD that demonstrates opening a sterile package and to store it on our school's Web server. This digitized segment would be accessible by only the registered students in the course and course faculty and support staff after password authentication. Credit for its use will, of course, be included.

It would be accessible via a link in the course content from August 1, 2008, through December 15, 2008.

If you do not control the copyright on all of the above-mentioned material, I would appreciate any contact information you can give me regarding the proper rights holder(s), including current

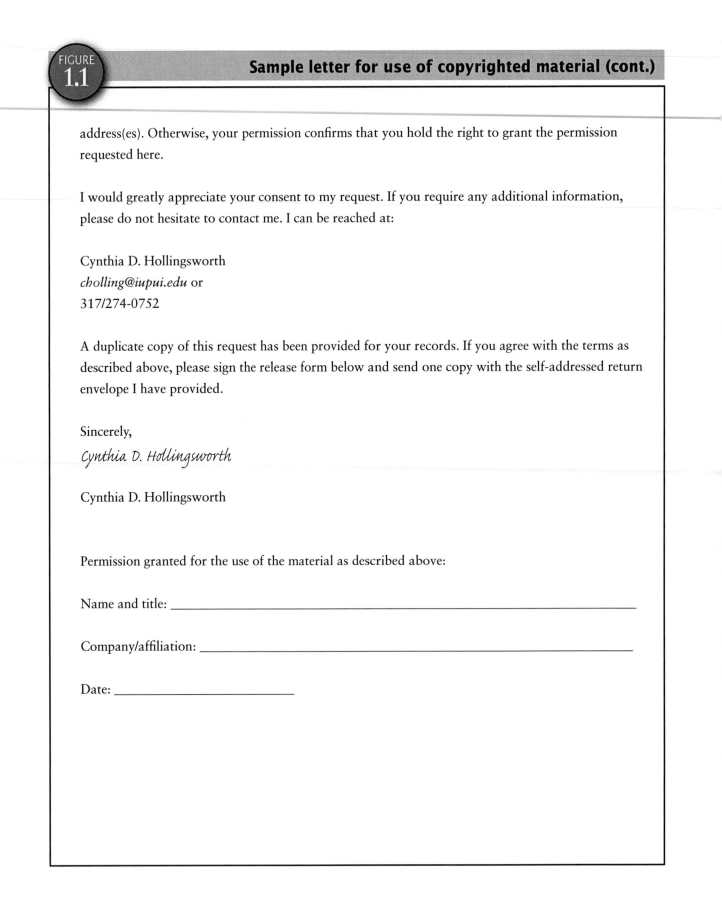

FIGURE 1.1 | **Sample letter for use of copyrighted material (cont.)**

address(es). Otherwise, your permission confirms that you hold the right to grant the permission requested here.

I would greatly appreciate your consent to my request. If you require any additional information, please do not hesitate to contact me. I can be reached at:

Cynthia D. Hollingsworth
cholling@iupui.edu or
317/274-0752

A duplicate copy of this request has been provided for your records. If you agree with the terms as described above, please sign the release form below and send one copy with the self-addressed return envelope I have provided.

Sincerely,

Cynthia D. Hollingsworth

Cynthia D. Hollingsworth

Permission granted for the use of the material as described above:

Name and title: _____

Company/affiliation: _____

Date: _____

Figure 1.2 summarizes the advantages and disadvantages of commercially prepared VHS and DVD audio/video technologies. You can see that, for the most part, they are fairly evenly matched—assuming that the media has already been purchased. Today, when purchasing media, institutions and educators would be wise to forego VHS media in favor of DVD technology in order to extend the useful life span of the investment.

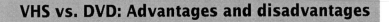

FIGURE 1.2

VHS vs. DVD: Advantages and disadvantages

Media	Advantages	Disadvantages
VHS/VCR	• Uses "teachable moments" • Loads easily • Transports easily • Works with remote control	• Consistent sound levels difficult to maintain • Occasional tape malfunctions • Replacement costs • Dated contents • Single source that meets all needs difficult to locate • Permission to use in distance education and distributed via networks required • Publisher-imposed stipulations on use
DVD	• Uses "teachable moments" • Loads easily • Transports easily • Works with remote control • Visual clarity improved over VHS quality	• Consistent sound levels difficult to maintain • Easily scratched or corrupted media • Replacement costs • Dated contents • Single source that meets all needs difficult to locate • Permission to use in distance education and distributed via networks required • Publisher-imposed stipulations on use

Figure 1.3 includes a form, used with permission from the Indiana University School of Nursing (IUSON), used by the Learning Laboratory when educators wish to preview educational videos. This completed document provides rationale for the video's use in meeting educational goals, summarizes the course and student demographics, and identifies the costs involved. After previewing the media, the faculty critiques its usefulness and recommends purchasing or returning the video and, if recommending purchase, prioritizes it. This background information, along with the expert advice of the faculty, gives the institution guidance in allocating resources while meeting the greatest needs of the school and learners. IUSON has offered this resource for use in your facilities and institutions.

FIGURE 1.3

Request form to preview educational videos

Indiana University School of Nursing Learning Laboratory:

Request to preview educational video form

Title of video: _____

Publisher: _____

Publisher address: _____

Publisher telephone number: _____

Purchase price: _____ Preview price: _____

Source of funding for purchase (department, grant, etc.):

Course to be used in:

Number of students:

Times per year to be used:

To be used in classroom: Learning lab: Clinical facility:

Complete after preview

Target audience:

Content (Summarize and comment on accuracy, topics included, appropriateness, presentation):

Describe how video supports course objectives:

Recommendation:

Purchase: Priority: (1–5; priority 1 is highest)

Return:

Faculty signature: _____

User-created media

Enter the new century and the advent of audio and video recordings that you can create in order to include the teaching and learning strategies you want to use to meet your educational goals.

PowerPoint

Software applications such as Microsoft PowerPoint® allow you to record voice narrations. These files are saved as Windows .wav files, which are embedded in the presentation file itself so that the recording can be played during the presentation. Recording narration is simple.

To create the narration, first find a quiet place. Although you may believe that your office is quiet, become aware of ambient noise, such as people walking and talking in the hallway outside the door, construction or traffic noise from outside, fans and blowers, unexpected chimes for incoming mail, ringing telephones, knocks on the door, and jewelry that may clatter against the desk or brush against the microphone. The best location for recording is quiet and does not have an echo—smaller rooms generally are best.

Other than the equipment, which we'll cover in the section on podcasts, the most important tool is a narration script. Do not rely on innate knowledge of your subject or the fact that you may have given a presentation on this topic numerous times. You will find that preparing a script or detailed outline makes editing much easier when you later rearrange the slides in the presentation, update text or presentation content, or make corrections.

TIP

First develop the presentation; then write the script.

New Technology in Nursing Staff Development

Because PowerPoint is unable to have a fluid narration that runs beneath multiple slides as they progress, isolate script components based on the presentation, allowing for breaks between slides. PowerPoint's speaker handout view provides a tool for creating your script. Notice in the samples shown in Figure 1.4 that you can type your narration directly on the handout page. Because you can adjust the size of the slide image and the text, you can easily include your script on that single slide. As you are recording, or later when reviewing your work, you have the visual cue of the slide itself. By isolating the text slide by slide, you can easily rerecord portions if you edit your presentation or flub a section as you record.

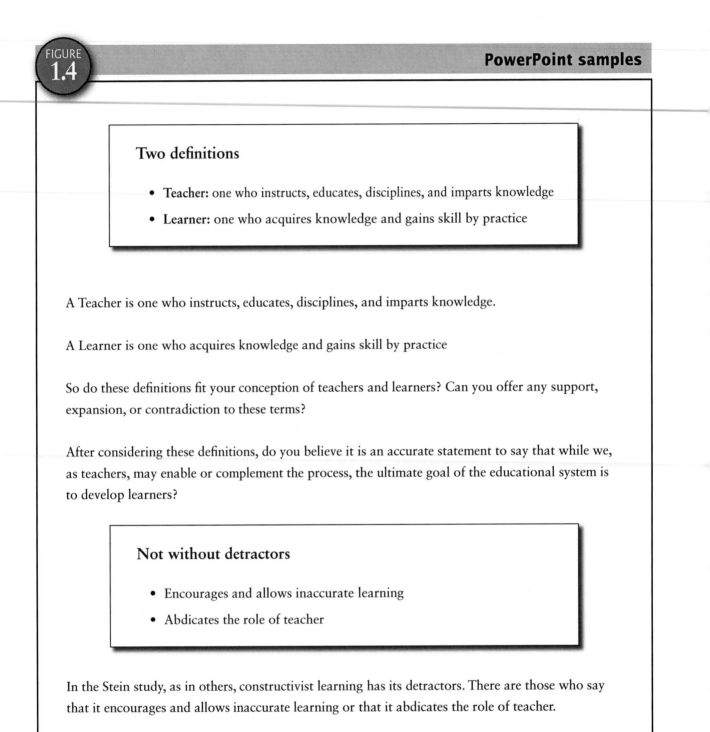

FIGURE
1.4

PowerPoint samples

Two definitions

- **Teacher:** one who instructs, educates, disciplines, and imparts knowledge
- **Learner:** one who acquires knowledge and gains skill by practice

A Teacher is one who instructs, educates, disciplines, and imparts knowledge.

A Learner is one who acquires knowledge and gains skill by practice

So do these definitions fit your conception of teachers and learners? Can you offer any support, expansion, or contradiction to these terms?

After considering these definitions, do you believe it is an accurate statement to say that while we, as teachers, may enable or complement the process, the ultimate goal of the educational system is to develop learners?

Not without detractors

- Encourages and allows inaccurate learning
- Abdicates the role of teacher

In the Stein study, as in others, constructivist learning has its detractors. There are those who say that it encourages and allows inaccurate learning or that it abdicates the role of teacher.

However, learners need guidance, and teachers will always be needed as role models, guiders of learning, and imparters of knowledge. But perhaps, the emphasis can be shifted to those who can benefit the most from learning: the learners.

Different versions of PowerPoint have slightly different controls and methods of access, but the principles are the same. For example, to record a narration in PowerPoint 2003, do the following:

1. Choose from the menu, SLIDE SHOW: Record Narration

2. After testing your microphone levels (which is highly recommended if this is your first narration attempt), click OK.

3. When your presentation begins, begin speaking. Be sure to pause at the end of the slide. Then transition to the next slide and resume speaking.

4. When you're finished, PowerPoint will prompt you to save or discard your audio file.

Recording a narration increases the total file size of your presentation, since the audio portion is stored along with the presentation slides, any images you have used, and any transitions you have added. Because PowerPoint presentations (particularly media-rich ones) can become quite large, it is better to create multiple presentations and show them in sequence than to create a single multi-megabyte presentation that will be slow to download or run.

One valuable software application you can add to your instructional technologies arsenal is called PowerShrink, published by Top Byte Labs (*www.powershrink.com*), which works with all Microsoft Office documents. This wonderful software can shrink your presentation by half or more, depending on the content in the presentation, and with no quality difference or change in functionality, formatting, or features. The under-$50 price provides a great resource for your library at a reasonable cost. A free trial allows you to test-drive the software to see whether it will work for you.

Video recorders/camcorders

Video recorders allow educators to record audio and video movies as well as design learning experiences wherein learners create their own A/V projects to build or demonstrate knowledge. A learning strategy used in community nursing courses has students travel into communities and create "windshield" surveys. Students videotape physical, geographical, and cultural components of neighborhoods and present their findings to their peers in class. For example, staff educators may create a video introducing their facility or a process that new staff nurses need to know. Educators can record guest speakers or experts in their field. Chief nursing officers may record a welcome to new staff nurses that can be played during orientation. The possibilities are as great as your imagination.

For less than $150, educators or learners can purchase a lightweight camcorder that plugs directly into the USB port in a computer (like a digital camera or a flash drive does). The Flip Video Ultra 4 (*www.theflip.com*) holds up to 60 minutes of recorded video, has a built-in flash, and records well in most light environments. It is easy to use and produces videos with a fair degree of quality. A flexible tripod—such as the Gorillapod Flexible Tripod from Joby (*www.joby.com*), which sells for less than $20—easily attaches to the video recorder. Its bendable, wrap-able legs allow you to position the recorder in a variety of positions in order to shoot focused, directed, non-blurry video.

Permissions

We would be remiss if we didn't mention the issues with privacy, permissions, and waivers. When we begin creating multimedia, it is easy to overlook the fact that sometimes the things we can do are not necessarily the things we should do, at least not without permission.

Creating a windshield survey and recording the buildings, yards, address signs, businesses, and people walking down the street in an anonymous fashion doesn't raise any privacy concerns, as there are no expectations of privacy on a public street. However, if an educator or learner wants to interview one of those individuals, then that individual has a right to refuse and to maintain his or her privacy. For this reason, it is important that prior to recording an interview, presentation, or speech or asking someone to participate with you in a recorded event, you must obtain a signed waiver/permission from that person. If the individual is a minor, then the permission of the parent or guardian should be obtained. Adolescents who are legally still minors but who are old enough to make decisions concerning their own privacy should be asked to sign a permission document on their own behalf in addition to the legally binding signature of a parent or guardian.

Figures 1.5, 1.6, 1.7, 1.8, and 1.9 include sample permission/waiver letters and copyright assignment samples, which can serve as models for your permission, waiver, and copyright assignment documents. They are used here with permission from the Copyright Management Center of Indiana University, located on the IUPUI campus.

 New Technology in Nursing Staff Development

FIGURE
1.5

Waiver for use of video likeness during a presentation

I, [insert full name], hereby grant permission to the [institution/organization/facility name] to record my likeness and presentation being delivered at [insert name of location] on [insert date], and to make that presentation available through the [institution/organization/facility's] networked resources for the purposes of distributing to [specifically delineate the purposes] offered by the [institution/organization/facility] for either academic or continuing education or in other presentations, marketing, and publications related to the teaching, learning, research, scholarship, and service missions of the school. I hereby release and discharge the videographer, his/her heirs, executors, assigns, and any designee (including any agency, client, broadcaster, periodical, or other publication) from any and all claims and demands arising out of or in connection with the use of such videos, film, or tape, including, but not limited to, any claims for defamation or invasion or privacy.

I understand that these rights should in no way restrict republication of the material in any other form by me or by others authorized by me.

[signed]
[typed name]
[date]

Waiver for use of video likeness (for a minor)

I, [insert full name], hereby grant permission to the [institution/organization/facility] to use the video likeness of my child, [insert full name], recorded at [insert name of location where video was recorded] on [insert date] by [insert name of videographer] and to make that recording available through the [institution/organization/facility's] networked resources for the purposes of distributing to [specifically delineate the purposes] offered by the [institution/organization/facility] for either academic or continuing education or in other presentations, marketing, and publications related to the teaching, learning, research, scholarship, and service missions of the school. I hereby release and discharge the videographer, his/her heirs, executors, assigns, and any designee (including any agency, client, broadcaster, periodical, or other publication) from any and all claims and demands arising out of or in connection with the use of such videos, film, or tape, including, but not limited to, any claims for defamation or invasion or privacy.

I understand that these rights should in no way restrict republication of the material in any other form by me or by others authorized by me.

[signed]
[typed name]
[date]

New Technology in Nursing Staff Development

FIGURE
1.7

Waiver for use of video likeness (for an adolescent)

I, [insert full name], hereby grant permission to the [institution/organization/facility] to use the video likeness of me recorded at [insert name of location where video was recorded] on [insert date] by [insert name of videographer], and to make that recording available through the [institution/organization/facility's] networked resources for the purposes of distributing to [specifically delineate the purposes] offered by the [institution/organization/facility] for either academic or continuing education or in other presentations, marketing, and publications related to the teaching, learning, research, scholarship, and service missions of the school. I hereby release and discharge the videographer, his/her heirs, executors, assigns, and any designee (including any agency, client, broadcaster, periodical, or other publication) from any and all claims and demands arising out of or in connection with the use of such videos, film, or tape, including, but not limited to, any claims for defamation or invasion or privacy.

I understand that this waiver in no way restricts republication of this video recording by me or by others authorized by me.

[signed]
[typed name]
[date]

I, [insert name], being the legal parent/guardian of [insert adolescent's name] being witness to the recording of the video likeness above described and witness to my child's informed consent, hereby consent according to the guidelines and stated purposes as outlined above.
[signed]
[typed name]
[date]

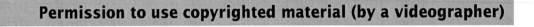

FIGURE
1.8

Permission to use copyrighted material (by a videographer)

I, [insert full name], am granting the [institution/organization/facility] permission to store, duplicate, broadcast, and make derivative copies of the video taken by me with permission from the parents/guardians of any minors and/or with permission of any adults in the videos on [insert date], for use in furtherance of the teaching, learning, research, and service missions of the [institution/organization/facility].

The requested permission extends to any future revisions and editions of any project, course, or the [institution/organization/facility] Web site or print publications, including nonexclusive world rights in all languages. Further, I understand that these rights should in no way restrict republication of the material in any other form by me or by others authorized by me. My signature on this document will also confirm that I own the copyright to the above-described material.

Permission granted for the use requested above:

[name]
[typed name]
[date]

FIGURE 1.9 — **Copyright assignment (by a staff or student as a "work-for-hire")**

In order to best facilitate the teaching and learning mission of the [institution/organization/facility] and to create a common framework of ownership for developing instructional materials as an integral part of the continuing education and academic educational programs, I agree that any copyrightable works that I may create within the scope of my service to [institution/organization/facility] in developing those instructional materials shall be regarded as "works made for hire" under the U.S. Copyright Act with ownership rights vesting in the [institution/organization/facility]. Should any such works not qualify as works made for hire, I hereby assign and transfer any copyright interests that I may have in and to such works to the [institution/organization/facility]. This agreement and its implementation will be subject to policies and procedures of the [institution/organization/facility] as may be in force from time to time regarding the ownership and management of intellectual property. I agree to cooperate with the [institution/organization/facility] to execute assignments, registrations, and any other documents related to the ownership of specific works created by me.

I retain the copyright to display such works in professional portfolios and other academic or professional activities such as derivative works and scholarly publications based on such works, provided that my actions do not conflict with the intended uses of the work by [institution/organization/facility] and do not conflict with the policies and procedures of [institution/organization/facility].

[name]
[typed name]
[date]

As mentioned previously, when discussing the sample to request permission, use the letters as samples and modify them as needed to fit your specific circumstances. Remember these specifics:

- Anyone you video or audio record should sign a waiver (or in the case of a minor, a parent/guardian should sign)

- If someone outside your organization is the videographer, then that individual needs to assign copyright ownership of the video to you and/or your institution, unless you have made other legally binding agreements.

- If someone (such as a student or staff member) employed by your organization is the videographer, then that work likely falls in the category of "work for hire." Nevertheless, a copyright agreement should be signed and filed for the protection of all parties.

Accessing media files

Once a video or audio file is created, accessing it is as simple as storing the file on a server and allowing users to download it. Often media files are stored on Web servers. This storage allows educators to distribute a URL to learners who then use a standard Web browser such as Microsoft Internet Explorer® or Mozilla Firefox® to retrieve the file. Learners need a player such as Real Player®, Windows Media Player®, or Apple Quicktime®, which are default installations on newer computers, in order to access the media. The specific player depends on the format of the media when it is created.

The disadvantage of this download method is that when a learner accesses the file, the entire file must be downloaded before playing can begin. And because media files—particularly video— can be quite large, it is often an arduous task to download unless the learner has a broadband connection such as cable or DSL.

An alternative storage is streaming media. Media must be stored on a server set up to process streaming, but the advantage is tremendous. When a file is accessed, rather than waiting until the entire file has been downloaded, streamed media begin playing while the download occurs.

Advantages and disadvantages

The advantages of these user-generated media are that they are relatively easy to create and generally cost-effective, especially when compared to commercial audio/video offerings. A major

 New Technology in Nursing Staff Development

disadvantage of these user-created projects is that the quality can be poor unless care is taken to ensure quality recordings. Educators should take care to ensure the highest quality; you don't want your professional image to appear with the quality of a jiggly, poorly lit home movie.

Finally, if a media file needs editing, you must either start from scratch and rerecord or have access to and knowledge of audio and/or video editing software, which takes the technological skill needs to a whole new dimension.

Podcasting and vodcasting

An iPod is a portable storage device created by Apple Computer (*www.apple.com*) in the early 2000s. The small gadget stores a large number of MP3 (an audio file format) audio files in order to create personalized playlists for a user. Advances in iPod technology now provide other file types besides MP3, which allows a broader range of audio and video to be accessed by the iPod.

The term "podcast" was first attributed to Ben Hammersley in 2004 (Van Orden) by combining the two terms "iPod" and "broadcast," since the Apple iPod was the most widely recognized brand of MP3 player. A podcast is, in its most basic form, an audio file. So what, you may ask, is the difference between the audio files we discussed previously and a podcast? The answer lies in how the user receives the file.

Podcasts are automatically downloaded to an MP3 player such as an iPod. When you find a resource containing something you are interested in, you can subscribe to it through a software application called a podcatcher. On a regular basis or when the file is updated, the podcatcher software gathers information about the updated file and sends it to your MP3 player or iPod. Some services send only headlines, whereas others retrieve complete files. The sources aren't necessarily only audio files but may be text or video formats as well. iPod users can create personalized multimedia service through mixing and matching music, speeches, newscasts, videos, headlines, weather, and personal viewpoints. Once downloaded to the player, users can start, stop, rewind, and replay as desired.

The advantage of this media versus streaming media (mentioned previously) is that learners are no longer tied to their computers to receive information but can receive it wherever they may be with their iPod or MP3 player.

"Great," you may say, "but where do I find these marvelous podcasts?"

When you're visiting Web sites, you may see small orange icons: one may look like sound waves, and the other may say RSS (which stands for Really Simple Syndication and is "geek speak" for a podcast subscription). These icons indicate that you can subscribe to a podcast. There are text-based feeds included on many Web sites, online journals, blogs (Web logs, or online journals), and news services. Apple iTunes (*www.apple.com/itunes*) works with iPods to allow users to subscribe to podcasts as well as to other services, such as the iTunes Store (to purchase music). Users also can subscribe to podcasts from personal computers through installed readers such as My Yahoo (*http://my.yahoo.com*), Google Reader (*www.google.com/reader*), and Bloglines (*www.bloglines.com*). Even Microsoft Outlook® has a RSS aggregator (another term for podcatcher) so that users can have their updates sent directly to their Outlook e-mail.

We've spent time talking about audio, but you may ask, "What about video?" That's a vodcast. A vodcast involves the same principles as a podcast, but instead of audio files being subscribed to and synchronized to your player, you subscribe to video feeds. Your computer can broadcast vodcasts through the players already installed on it, or if you have a newer model iPod, it can receive and play vodcasts.

Creating your first podcast

As we discussed previously in the section on recording PowerPoint narration, preparing for your podcast is important. Although some people may choose to create their podcast by speaking extemporaneously, most people—particularly educators—will have a better, more professional end product if the podcast is created while speaking from a script or at least a detailed outline. As with PowerPoint narrations, the choice of location is very important so that the broadcast is of the highest possible quality.

Be prepared to spend considerable time preparing for and recording your first podcast; some estimates range from two to four times the length of the podcast broadcast itself. It does get easier as you go along, but learning about and becoming comfortable with a new technology— especially one in which you're not only the director but the main actor—takes most people some time to become accustomed to.

Don't try to develop podcasts for your complete lecture series the first time. Start with something fun, like a description of Aunt Millie's 75th birthday party!

After creating your first podcast, listen to it, and have others listen to it. Listen for unexpected noises that you will want to control during recording sessions. Also note whether you are prone to using filler words such as "um" or "er," or need practice in modulating your voice pitch. After you've become somewhat accustomed to the sound of your own voice, create a podcast of light material, such as a welcome to your course or lecture, or an explanation to accompany a series of photographs. Then you'll be ready to tackle the heavy-duty topics.

Basic computer needs include:

- Windows (2000 or XP) or a Macintosh (OS 9 or 10)

- Minimum of 512 MB RAM

- Plenty of hard drive space (2–3 gigabytes is recommended for storage)

- Sound card—Creative Technology's Soundblaster Audigy® is a good one

- Headset/microphone—Logitech®, Plantronics®, and Labtech® are good equipment brands and cost $20–$40

- Sound editing/capture software (Audacity—*http://audacity.sourceforge.net*—is free)

With the Audacity software and sound card installed on your computer, your headset with microphone, your quiet ensured, and your script in front of you, you're ready to create your first podcast. Audacity contains a simple tutorial and help files to guide you through the individual steps at *http://audacityteam.org.*

Copyright

To really spiff up a podcast, educators may decide to include music in the background or to transition between segments of the podcast. Keep in mind that copyright prohibits the use of others' work without permission. Just because there is a purchased CD sitting on the shelf doesn't give the podcaster (i.e., a person who creates podcasts) permission to use "Free Bird" or "The Flight of the Bumblebee" in a podcast.

Fortunately, there are many music resources on the Web that are created for the purpose of using in podcast development. One you might try is Garageband (*www.garageband.com*).

Educational strategies

Strategies for using A/V technologies are as varied as the educators who choose to use them. A/V instructional technologies can:

- Supplement educator-delivered material

- Reach learners with a variety of learning styles

- Facilitate learning at the time and place of the learner's choosing

- Provide remediation opportunities

- Present guest experts from a distance

- Provide supplemental and enrichment opportunities for learners

- Demonstrate difficult concepts in a variety of ways

Financial considerations

A/V technologies, as with any instructional technologies, can be costly, but through the diligence of the educator reviewing the products; discussing options with publishers, vendors, and instructional technologies staff members; and looking at the amortization costs throughout the useful life span of the technology, these costs can be managed.

In budget planning, educators can expect to pay a couple to several hundred dollars for instructional videos, which often have a life span of several years; however, once purchased, there are no more fees. Getting set up with audio and video recording can be accomplished for a few hundred dollars unless you want a full-fledged sound recording studio and high-end video editing capabilities. The software tools identified in this chapter ranged from $20 to about $200.

The key, as with any major purchase, is to do your research. Talk to others who have walked the path you are preparing to tread, and be certain to talk with your network staff. Ask vendors for samples, trial periods, in-house demonstrations, and available technology support following purchase. Start with quality equipment that you can add to, but don't try to purchase everything that's available until you know whether these tools and these strategies are ones that work for you, your learners, and your learning objectives.

Evaluating your options

Previously, we discussed general advantages and disadvantage of a variety of A/V technologies, but you may be wondering, "That's great for them, but will it work for my organization? How do I convince 'the powers that be?' And how do I get busy, overworked nurses to actually use it?" The conclusion of this chapter will give you some options and strategies to consider.

Deciding on the right technology

Change means resistance. It means taking time to make adjustments in order to incorporate it into the mainstream. To evaluate whether podcasting, vodcasting, and other A/V technologies will be effective for you and your organization, ask yourself the following questions:

- **Do you understand how your educational offerings will be used by your intended audience?** If you enter any new educational arena without being able to address this issue, then you will probably have better odds at a casino than success with the technology. For example, nurses may believe that podcasts would be wonderful because it would allow them to complete mandatory training during commute time; however, HR will say, "No way. You have to complete mandatory on-the-clock training because, otherwise, we'll have to pay overtime."

- **Are you able to veer away from other technological teaching methods?** Your technology staff may encourage the staff educator to develop audio training since one of the goals is consistency across training; however, you may know that there is no way for a busy nurse to listen to an audio session at a relatively public computer on the floor.

Technology is not the answer; it's a means to a goal. First determine the goal you need to meet, identify your audience and their needs, and then consider technology options that will help you to achieve those goals for that audience.

Justifying your resources

With new technologies, in particular, it's better to start small and get some successes under your belt rather than deploy your entire educational program as podcasts or vodcasts just to learn that there are insurmountable obstacles.

For example, you may determine that vodcasting would be a great solution to refresh nurses' memories about infrequently used equipment; nurses can see the equipment in front of them and view a demonstration of basic functions to jog their memories of when they were trained on the equipment with their preceptor. Check to see whether the manufacturer has developed such a vodcast. If so, check with your representative to see whether the company will offer it free of charge or at a nominal fee for a short trial period. If so, you may be able to identify a technology savvy nurse who owns an iPod who would be willing to test the vodcast. This will provide you with data of what works, what problems arise, and how much interest it may generate among other staff members. The realization of these solutions is crucial to justifying the time and money (even if minimal) that is needed to institute these new A/V technologies.

Obtaining administrative buy-in

Once you can demonstrate that the technology is reliable and that the education plan is feasible, you can begin to enlist the assistance of "early adopters" who want to try new ways of learning. Success breeds success. Start small and build a program. Don't try to get administrator buy-in of new ideas without being able to show that you have a plan and that the plan works. Consider applying for a grant to purchase players, cameras, and headsets for podcasts, vodcasts, and A/V needs; many professional organizations, and government entities such as the National Institutes of Health, have technology/educational grants.

When you approach administrators, you need to be able to demonstrate that the use of these A/V technologies is not a "flash in the pan" but a viable way to deliver education to already over-worked staff members. The best way to do that is to walk into a meeting with evidence that it can work at a reasonable cost and address an identified problem effectively. Make sure to demonstrate through numbers and data that moving to this new technology would be a beneficial move for your organization.

Obtaining staff buy-in

For staff acceptance, you must demonstrate that the new technology isn't an addition to their workload but a resolution of a problem. Confront the apprehension that change brings with documented evidence that this is a realistic solution, not an additional problem to be overcome. And realize that this way of learning will not be for every nurse in every situation; it is simply another tool in the educator's arsenal of tools.

Conclusion

Audio and video can enhance or detract from education and should be used thoughtfully and for a purpose beyond "the cool factor." This chapter has given you a bird's-eye view of A/V technology of recent years, as well as some advantages and disadvantages of the various technologies. New instructional strategies can be intimidating, but start with baby steps and soon you'll be running to the nearest A/V technology with grand ideas for enhancing your educational offerings, making learning accessible to a wide variety of learners, and having fun!

References

Audacity. Source Forge. Retrieved July 17, 2008, from *http://audacity.sourceforge.net/*.

Bloglines. IAC Search & Media. Retrieved July 17, 2008, from *www.bloglines.com/*.

Creating a simple voice and music Podcast with Audacity. Audacity. Retrieved June 22, 2008, from *http://audacityteam.org/wiki/index.php?title=Creating_a_simple_voice_and_music_Podcast_with_Audacity*.

Flip Video Ultra. Retrieved July 17, 2008, from *www.theflip.com/store/Product.aspx?CID=F2*.

Garageband. iLike, Inc. Retrieved July 17, 2008, from *www.garageband.com/htdb/index.html*.

Google Reader. Google. Retrieved July 17, 2008, from *www.google.com/accounts/ServiceLogin?hl=en&nui=1&service=reader&continue=http%3A%2F%2Fwww.google.com%2Freader*.

Gorillapod Flexible Tripod. Joby. Retrieved July 17, 2008, from *www.joby.com/*.

Headsets. Plantronics. Retrieved July 17, 2008, from *http://plantronics.com/north_america/en_US/?_requestid=1632375*.

Headsets. Labtec. Retrieved July 17, 2008, from *www.labtec.com/index.cfm/gear/listing/AMR/EN,crid=8*.

Internet Headsets. Logitech. Retrieved July 17, 2008, from *www.logitech.com/index.cfm/webcam_communications/internet_headsets_phones/&cl=us,en*.

iPod. Apple Computer. Retrieved July 17, 2008, from *www.apple.com/*.

iTunes. Apple Computer. Retrieved July 17, 2008, from *www.apple.com/itunes*.

Model Permissions Letters. (2008, April 16). Copyright Advisory Office, Columbia University Libraries/Information Services. Retrieved July 17, 2008, from *www.copyright.columbia.edu/model-permissions-letters*.

My Yahoo. Yahoo! Inc. Retrieved July 17, 2008, from *http://p22.my.mud.yahoo.com/s/about/rss/*.

Request to Preview Educational Video Form. Indiana University School of Nursing.

PowerShrink. Top Byte Labs. Retrieved July 17, 2008, from *www.powershrink.com*.

Soundblaster Audigy. Creative Technology, Inc. Retrieved July 17, 2008, from *www.soundblaster.com/*.

Van Orden, J. (n.d.). The History of Podcasting. Citing The Guardian, February 12, 2004. Retrieved June 22, 2008, from *www.how-to-podcast-tutorial.com/history-of-podcasting.htm*.

Wallener, D. (n.d.). What is an iPod? Retrieved June 22, 2008, from *www.wisegeek.com/what-is-an-ipod.htm*.

Webcasts and Web conferencing

Webcasts, podcasts, simulcasts, TV show casts, casts for broken bones ... too many casts! What's an educator supposed to make of them all? Well, Chapter 1 discusses podcasts, and there's little we can do to improve TV show casts or fix casts on broken bones (although some nurses are good at that), so that leaves us to discussions of Webcasts and simulcasts. We'll even throw in Web conferences just to round things out. Jump on in—the water's fine!

Webcasts

Although the terms "Webcast," "Web conference," and "video conference" often are used synonymously, there are distinct differences between the three.

A Webcast is a broadcast via the Web. It originates at a single source and may be accessed by a single recipient or by multiple recipients using Web browsers. A Webcast is a one-way transmission, meaning that the recipients are passive receivers of the information. Simulcasts are special types of Webcasts. You may have noticed announcements during television news broadcasts indicating that they are being simulcast on a particular radio frequency or at a specific Web address.

This means that you can receive the broadcast at that radio frequency or Web address as it is being delivered on the television.

Webcasts can be live or streamed. Streamed Webcasts (meaning that you can begin watching the recording as it is being downloaded to the computer) are recorded during live presentations and stored on a special server, where they can be accessed for viewing later. Although there are no particular requirements, other than a computer, video cards, and sound cards (which are standard on most new computers), and an Internet connection for viewers of Webcasts, those creating Webcasts must have access to:

- Sufficient upload bandwidth rate (at least 100 KBps [kilobytes per seconds])—no dial-up! If you're considering becoming a Webcaster and want to test your upload speed, visit *www.speakeasy.net/speedtest* for a free test.

- A streaming server that will capture the audio and video, then encode and transmit the presentation.

- A Web server that will act as a portal for those accessing the Webcast, both real-time and any archived versions.

Because a Webcast is a live presentation (even though it may be delayed access), Webcasters will find it helpful to have a network support person present during creation of the Webcast in order to troubleshoot any problems that may arise.

An excellent resource for learning to be a Webcaster and honing your skills is the Webcast Academy (*www.webcastacademy.net*). The Academy is, by its own definition, "a hands-on, collaborative training center for people interested in learning how to produce and host live, interactive webcasts." There are many freely accessible resources on the site.

Web conferencing

The terms "Web conferencing" and "video conferencing" often are used synonymously; however, although both are interactive technologies and may be point-to-point (one-to-one interaction) or multi-point (one-to-many or many-to-many interactions), video conferencing uses a foundation of telecommunication technologies, whereas Web conferencing uses the Web. Both types of technology allow interaction via two-way video and audio transmissions simultaneously. As more users subscribe to services allowing greater transmission speeds, such as broadband and DSL, the capabilities of the two technologies become more similar—hence the interchangeability of the terms for most people.

Video conferencing

Polycom (*www.polycom.com*) is probably one of the most well-known video conferencing products, and others include PicturePhone, Inc. (*www.picturephone.com*) and WebEx (*www.webex. com)*. These video conferencing systems are installed at many educational and professional institutions, but many now are being supplanted by Web conferencing such as Adobe Acrobat Connect® (formerly Breeze). The system uses telecommunications lines to connect sites in the conference. Participants in the conference instruct their video conferencing unit to call a specified number to make the conference connection. Any participating site can be either a sending location or a receiving location.

Many video conferencing installations have a teaching station equipped with a computer attached to a projector and a document camera. System controls allow the educator or presenter to display information on the computer or to place documents or "overhead transparencies" on the document camera to display to the participants. Voice-activated or manually operated cameras allow the individual speaking to be displayed to other conference participants. All participants can view the others on the remote video display.

Web conferencing overview

Web conferencing first became widely available in the late 90s and functions in much the same manner as video conferencing, except that access is made through standard Web browsers. An individual or organization hosting a Web conference publishes a URL for attendees to access. Generally, the same URL is used for live access as well as for archived access. Some popular Web conferencing systems include Adobe Acrobat Connect (formerly Breeze) (*www.adobe.com/ products/acrobatconnect*), Elluminate (*www.elluminate.com*), TelSpan (*www.telspan.com*), and WebEx (*www.webex.com*).

Another conferencing resource that is quickly gaining in popularity is Skype (*www.skype.com*) due to its free or minimal cost (depending on the services), easy installation, and simple functioning. Skype members can "skype" other members using a computer, Web camera, and headset.

Calls are free of charge. These one-to-one Web conferences work like the videophones that our science fiction movies used to demonstrate. You also can conference with Skype; however, with more than two participants, you lose the video component. With the purchase of Skype minutes, this communications technology can even be used to make calls to land-based telephones.

Essential components

When researching which Web conferencing technology is right for you, look for these essential components:

- **Screen sharing:** This function allows the participant to share his or her computer desktop. This causes the display on the other participants' computers to show what the shared desktop looks like, including windows opening and closing, mouse movement, and actions being taken within the applications. This function is perfect for demonstrating application functionality. For example, an instructor could demonstrate how to form an appropriate function in Excel, add a transition to a PowerPoint slide, access a learning management system, post a threaded discussion forum, or run a statistical report.

- **Polling:** This survey function allows presenters to add "on-the-fly" questions and radio responses. As participants respond, the results are tabulated instantaneously and displayed to all participants. For example, a presenter might ask, "Have you ever participated in a Web conference before?" or "Does your institution own a SimMan?" or "Do you anticipate your institution requiring preceptors to be at least master's prepared?" This feature allows presenters to target specific audience components or to shift the focus of a presentation during the presentation itself for a richer learning experience.

- **Whiteboards:** This functionality mimics a classroom whiteboard, allowing a participant to use a computer mouse as a marker. Presenters can either control the whiteboard or open the access for participants to also use the function. Here's an example: Many learners find math difficult; for many, learning math online is even more problematic. The benefit of an educator writing the equation step-by-step (which participants see as they are developed on-screen) while explaining the sequence (which participants hear through the audio broadcast) clarifies the process, providing a learning environment suited to both aural and visual learners. If the educator also allows the participants to use the whiteboard function, then kinesthetic learners also benefit by being able to include their own examples.

- **Chat:** The ability to have an ongoing chat during a presentation is critical. Participants can pose questions to the presenters, include anecdotal information, and share Web URLs. Presenters clarify points, expand on points of interest to the participants, and request participant feedback. With large numbers of participants, though, a lively chat also necessitates a moderator. As the presenter speaks, the moderator can watch the chat room and feed questions or remarks to the presenter.

- **Application sharing:** As an extension of the shared desktop, application sharing actually allows participants to jointly control an application to create a collaborative document.

Technical requirements

For participants in a Web conference, these are the optimal technical requirements:

- **Computer:** Pentium 4, 2.4 GHz or faster, with 1 GB or more of RAM (minimal components: Pentium, 1 GHz speed, and 512 MB of RAM)

- **Operating System:** Windows 2000 or XP; Mac OS X

- **Internet connection:** Broadband (DLS or cable) with a connection speed of 256 KBps—both download and upload speed—with little latency (latency is the delay between an occurrence and when you are aware of the occurrence). Note: Satellite connections have too much latency and are not effective Web-conferencing solutions.

- **Audio/video:** USB camera and headset (or headphones and a separate microphone, although audio quality seems to be better with a headset); Logitech (*www.logitech.com*) and Plantronics (*http://plantronics.com*) sell products that are reasonably priced and provide quality sound.

- **Web browser:** Firefox 2.0® or Internet Explorer 7.0®

Solutions and benefits

Web conferencing is an ideal solution for many reasons:

- If you have ever attempted to coordinate the schedules of busy educators or other professionals, you'll know it is nearly impossible. How much simpler to get them all together if they don't have to all be together!

> **TIP**
>
> You will also find it beneficial to have a Flash player, version 6.0 or higher, installed on your computer, since many Web sites use this technology for interactive components.

- Have an out-of-town interviewee? Need to have faculty from another state participate in a dissertation defense? You can avoid travel expenses.

- Do you want a guest lecturer for your seminar next month, but she happens to be in Europe at a conference? Have her present a Web conference to your class.

- Does your grant review committee have questions? Do administrators at various locations of your institution have questions about the draft proposal? No need to swap e-mail messages; talk face-to-face.

Webinars

A Webinar is a special type of Web conferencing. This Web-based seminar uses Web conferencing to present a topic to participants. Often, this is a one-way Web presentation, with participants watching a demonstration using their Web browsers and participating through a telephone connection. Here's a sample scenario:

A school of nursing's continuing education (CE) office offers a three-course series on beginning staff education. Hospital A, which is on the opposite side of the United States from the nursing school's CE office, is considering enrolling several new staff educators in the Web-based series of courses because it is more cost-effective than developing their own orientation for the didactic content, freeing up their orientation time for hospital-specific training. The CE office arranges a Webinar and notifies the staff educator of the URL and the call-in telephone number. At the agreed-upon time, the staff educator, at his own office computer, accesses the URL and telephones the CE office. While sitting in his office, the staff educator can watch a demonstration of accessing the learning management system, see components of the course, and watch as learning activities are demonstrated. At the same time, the staff educator and the CE staff can discuss the course, ask and answer questions, and target the demonstration according to the needs of the staff educator.

All of this isn't to say that Web conferencing is the ideal solution for every situation, of course. Participants must ensure that their computer has at least the minimum recommended configuration or participation becomes frustrating. Some people find it too easy to attempt to multitask while participating in a conference, leading to decreased benefit of participating. Webcasters who present to an empty room often find it difficult to envision a rapt audience and to generate the enthusiasm that they would when presenting to a live audience. Also consider time zone differences when scheduling Web conferences if the audience and presenter are to be live rather than accessing an archive.

Tips for on-camera presenters

We'll conclude this chapter with tips for on-camera presenters. We hope that these tips guide effective preparation and presentation practices whether the camera is in an electronic classroom or a broadcast room or a video conferencing environment or via a Webcam. The tips below are divided, rather loosely, into the following categories: presentation preparation, document preparation, your presentation appearance, audience engagement, and delivering the presentation.

Presentation preparation

Remember watching the evening news and seeing the anchor look into the wrong camera? If there are multiple cameras available, such as a local and a remote during a video conference, make certain you know which camera is sending a signal to the remote audience and which camera is sending a signal to your local site. Otherwise, you're not making eye contact with your audience—and they're wondering who you're watching!

Video conferences are scheduled to begin and end at exact times in order to maintain busy broadcast schedules. Some systems come on for testing approximately 10 minutes before the scheduled presentation time, and most systems shut off without warning when the conference time is complete. Therefore, it is important that you, as the presenter, are in your seat and prepared to begin right on time—and preferably before.

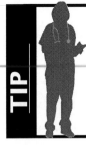

Be sure to rehearse your presentation carefully in order to complete it before being cut off. Remember, video conferencing doesn't give you a five-minute warning; it simply stops in preparation for the next scheduled conference. You may find it helpful to designate someone at your location as your timekeeper. This individual could signal you when you are nearing the end of your scheduled broadcast time.

Because habits such as continually clearing your throat, saying "um" or "uh," or nervous giggling or shuffling are enhanced on camera, consider rehearsing your presentation by videotaping it and reviewing it prior to your on-camera presentation. Another option is to schedule, if time and schedule permits, a practice conference. Have a trusted colleague there with you to watch during a live presentation or to review an archived session. Don't rely on your own judgment—we are generally our own worst critics.

Because cameras and microphones will pick up any extraneous noise, do not play with change or keys in your pocket, drum your fingers on the table, or shuffle papers during a conference, and don't clink ice in a cup or slurp through a straw or crunch on a snack when the camera isn't watching.

When using systems in which the cameras automatically change to the last site (or person) to make a noise, it will help for you to alleviate some of the camera refocusing during the conference by defining camera presets to "lock in" camera shots on specific speakers or groups of participants. Presets can be established before the conference, then during the presentation simply choose the preset you wish the camera to move to. It will also be helpful to remind all participants to mute their microphones when not speaking. In systems in which sound activates the cameras, sideline conversations and unexpected noises cause the cameras to turn and refocus.

Document preparation

The following tips will help when creating your presentation:

- Create documents with a landscape orientation (more wide than tall).

- Try to make all your visuals the same size so that you can pre-focus the document camera before the presentation.

 New Technology in Nursing Staff Development

- Use large lettering (no less than 36-point type, greater if the receiving site may have more than six participants) on visuals and a sans serif font (such as Verdana, Arial, Helvetica, or Geneva).

- Use no more than two different fonts in your presentation visuals.

- Use italicized text sparingly, if at all, since it can be more difficult to read.

- Place no more than four lines per page, six words per line on documents, centered vertically on the page to allow ample margins.

- Leave at least 1.5-inch margins, and allow white space between lines of type.

- Light blue paper with black, bold text reduces glare from the lights and still provides high contrast for easier viewing.

- Create documents with high contrast between paper and text. The standard black text on white paper is still extremely effective.

- Keep the background on documents a solid color without gradients or patterns.

- If you want to use color for emphasis, bright yellow (think of the color that children color sunshine!) on "true blue" works very well.

- Avoid combinations of low-contrast colors, such as blue on green or orange on yellow.

- Avoid red-green color combinations for the benefit of those who are color blind.

- In general, avoid using red because it tends to "bleed," leaving text looking unclear.

- Keep in mind that monitor quality varies from site to site. Test color combinations at different color settings during development to ensure that all of your audience will see an effective visual.

- Thin lines can appear to waiver on camera. If you use lines in your visuals, make sure that they are at least three points or wider.

- Avoid displaying complex or dense diagrams on the document camera. If a complex diagram is essential, consider mailing, e-mailing, or faxing it to each remote site so they can review a hard copy, or making it available as a download from a Web site and simply providing the URL (preferably beforehand if it's something the participants need to understand before or during the presentation).

- When possible, provide a hard copy (faxed or mailed) of the agenda to each participating location prior to the presentation.

- If you send handouts to the viewing locations before the presentation, make sure that each handout is arranged in the order of presentation so that your audience can take notes and follow along.

Your presentation appearance

Your appearance matters, so follow these tips:

- The best colors to wear are moderate hued blues, greens, and purples.

- Avoid wearing black (very harsh under the camera), white (glares), and red (bleeds) clothing.

- Colors appear darker than they really are, so navy blue, for example, will look black on camera.

- Avoid wearing clothing with plaids, checks, and bold prints.

- Avoid jewelry that catches the glare of the lights, may reflect light, or cause noise that the cameras may pick up.

Audience engagement

For the most effective presentation, your audience needs to be engaged, so pay attention to these best practices:

- Conduct a roll call at the beginning of the broadcast so that everyone knows what sites are participating and periodically in the first five to seven minutes if you have late arrivals.

- Introduce yourself.

- To maintain "eye contact" with your audience, look into the sending camera as well as occasionally making eye contact with any audience in the room with you.

 New Technology in Nursing Staff Development

- Encourage participants to preface remarks with identification such as, "This is Cindy from Indianapolis."

- When possible, focus the camera on the person speaking.

- To engage your audience when they are scattered among several locations, plan to poll each site, by name, at various times during the conference for questions or comments in order to engage the audience at that site (most won't feel comfortable interrupting otherwise).

- Consider planting some questions at each site in order to start the conversation, in case it doesn't seem to initiate spontaneously.

- Always repeat the question or summarize a comment for the benefit of participants who may not have heard the comment and for the benefit of the archived conference.

- Allow sufficient time for responses from the various sites; it may take a moment for a participant at another site to get off mute and begin speaking when she/he wants to ask a question or make a comment.

- Be assertive in not allowing a member of your audience to dominate the presentation.

- Be assertive in summarizing a particular segment and moving on in order to keep on schedule.

- Remember not to ignore the live audience in the room with you because you're trying to be aware of the audience at other viewing sites.

- Try to build in time for a short question-and-answer session at the end of each module in your presentation.

Delivering the presentation

During the presentation, it's important not to get sidetracked, so prepare in advance by following these tips:

- Broadcast rooms are often equipped with microphones to pick up audio signals. Some rooms have ceiling mounted microphones; others have microphones on the tables. Decide before the broadcast whether you will stand or sit during your presentation. In rooms equipped with table microphones, if you decide to deliver your presentation standing, you may need to wear a lapel microphone in order to have the sound of your voice picked up by the system. In rooms equipped with ceiling microphones, you may need to project your voice upward in order for the sound of your voice to be adequately broadcast (but don't watch the ceiling!).

- Place a "title" sheet on the document camera identifying your presentation and location before the beginning of the presentation. When each site comes on air, your site will be identified to them.

- Allow a couple of minutes at the very beginning of the broadcast for a settling-in period to get participants seated and on air before beginning your presentation, but don't hesitate to call the meeting to order with the audience you have or you won't finish during the allotted broadcast.

- Introduce yourself.

- Provide an agenda on the document camera at the beginning of the presentation that includes the broadcast time. Doing so lets each member of the audience be aware of the focus of the presentation and the amount of time available.

- If you take a break during your presentation, place a note on the document camera that says, "Break. Back at ... " If you handwrite the note, make sure that it is in dark ink, large letters, and legible handwriting.

- Many video cameras are activated by sound; be careful to keep your site on mute when you are not speaking.

- Remind your audience that each site should keep their site on mute when someone at that site is not speaking; otherwise, the site making the noise will become the sending site and you will see the cameras jump to that location.

- Remind your audience that when their site is on mute, they must turn mute off before asking a question or making a comment.

- Speak with a well-modulated voice and enunciate clearly.

New Technology in Nursing Staff Development

- Consider recruiting someone to assist, who can operate any document cameras and control tablets, which will make it easier to deliver your presentation.

- Be careful not to leave the same image on the monitor for long periods of time. Vary the image on the monitor by allowing (or requiring) participation from each site, by using the document camera, and by using various camera views.

- When you continue to speak as you are displaying something on the document camera, you become a disembodied voice. Keep the camera focused on the document camera only as long as necessary, and then come back on camera.

- Remain aware of the time remaining in your presentation. You may find it helpful to enlist the assistance of a participant at your location, who can give you a sign at the 15-, 10-, and five-minute marks.

- You should begin winding down a few minutes before the scheduled ending time. Use this time to summarize the presentation's key points and to make sure that the audience knows how to contact you for further information or clarification.

- Have your presentation files available on disk or on overhead transparencies in the event that the network goes down.

- Build in extra time during the presentation to manipulate the mouse and recover from technical glitches.

- If you plan to use the Internet, you may find it helpful to have saved key document files on your local workstation and view them as local files, rather than via a live connection.

- Be aware that transmission noise may come across the system during your presentation; don't let it distract you.

- If you have requested that your presentation be recorded, remember that even if your location is on mute and the other sites can not hear you, any noise or conversation at your location will be recorded on the tape.

- Remember that viewing a video presentation is not the same as watching TV. Keep in mind that when a participant from another site is speaking, the camera may well still be on you. Looking inattentive, bored, or otherwise uninterested will reflect poorly on you and be displayed clearly across all the viewing sites.

Financial considerations

For educators, the financial considerations of Webcasts and Web conferencing vary tremendously on whether the infrastructure pieces are already in place or not. For example, if servers already exist that can stream Webcasts and store archived broadcasts, then the educator's financial outlays are relatively small. For under $100, an educator can purchase a headset and Web camera, allowing him or her to broadcast from his or her office.

In a similar vein, individual educators are not generally willing or able—both financially and technologically—to set up and run their own video conferencing setups but instead must rely on institutional resources. If you're an educator who wishes to "dip your toe" into the Webcast/Web conferencing pool with minimal financial costs, then Skype is the way to start. With the cost of a pair of Webcams and headsets, and a colleague who will agree to join the fun, you can practice conferencing with no additional cost, since Skype is a free service.

Evaluating your options

We've discussed the good and bad of Webcasts and Web conferencing, but how do you decide whether they're right for you?

Deciding on the right technology

One of your first considerations in using these technologies is your environment. You need a quiet place in which to create a Webcast so participants can easily discuss topics out loud during a conference. They are some of the most cost-effective technologies discussed in this book. They are also learner-and educator-friendly with minimal training time being required to get up to speed.

One of the biggest challenges for using this type of technology is time variations. Since (with the exception of archived broadcasts) these sessions occur in real time, time zone differences have to be factored into the equation. Additionally, educators may find that it helps learners to feel comfortable with these technologies by giving them an opportunity to experience aspects of Web conferencing before involving them in classroom training. For example, use the first few minutes of class to allow your nurses to view a noneducational Web conference. You could also review a mock conference script to allow them to get accustomed to the format. Giving your nurses this chance to familiarize themselves with the technology prior to training will help them ease into the set up.

New Technology in Nursing Staff Development

Justifying your resources

When justifying resources that are necessary for implementing Webcasts and Web conferences, remember that this form of education has many rewards and does not require great shifts in learning on the part of the student from traditional classroom training, particularly when coupled with desktop sharing applications. Be sure to recognize and point out these rewards, such as:

- The advantage of having the educator and student not have to be at the same location in order for training to take place

- The ability to avoid travel expenses by having out-of-town participants present a Web conference

- The capability to discuss projects (such as grant proposals) with administrators face-to-face via a Web conference rather than over the phone or through e-mail

These benefits are key to justifying this type of technology.

Obtaining administrative buy-in

Two of the primary motivators for administrators for these technologies are the savings of time and money. As the costs of Webcasts and Web conferences are minimal, you will be able to show your administrators that the benefits that we have outlined in this chapter are worth the low costs. Additionally, you can demonstrate that this training method is an excellent way to save valuable teaching time. Rather than having to travel to meetings or classes, with the use of a computer, cost-effective headset and camera, the education can take place on-site, even if other learners and educators are elsewhere.

Obtaining staff buy-in

Some learners first find it disconcerting to be on camera, but most quickly become involved in the interaction and forget that there's a camera involved. Make sure you ease their possible stage fright as you look to obtain staff member buy-in. Emphasize that these technologies are great for learners who need the face-to-face interaction since they can see the other participants. At the same time, it works in many ways for those learners who are looking for distance education since the participants can still be geographically separate.

Conclusion

When you first begin to video or Web conference, you may well feel intimidated by the technology and cameras, ... and that's okay. Most people are not comfortable in front of a camera or in hearing their own recorded voice. With time, it will get easier, and these are wonderful technologies. Use your imagination; let the possibilities soar and be sure to have fun.

References

Acrobat Connect Pro. (n.d.). Adobe, Inc. Retrieved July 20, 2008, from *www.adobe.com/resources/breeze/*.

Breeze/Web Conferencing. (n.d.). Indiana University School of Nursing. Retrieved July 20, 2008, from *http://nursing.iupui.edu/students/breeze_technologies.shtml*.

Elluminate. (n.d.). Retrieved July 20, 2008, from *www.elluminate.com*.

Flash (n.d.). Adobe, Inc. Retrieved July 17, 2008, from *www.adobe.com/shockwave/download/download. cgi?P1_Prod_Version=shockwaveFlash*.

Headsets. Plantronics. Retrieved July 17, 2008, from *http://plantronics.com/north_america/en_US/?_ requestid=1632375*.

Internet Headsets. Logitech. Retrieved July 17, 2008, from *www.logitech.com/index.cfm/webcam_ communications/internet_headsets_phones/&cl=us,en*.

Online surgical and healthcare video and webcasts. (n.d.). ORlive. Retrieved July 20, 2008, from *www.or-live.com/*.

PicturePhone. (n.c.). Retrieved July 20, 2008, from *www.picturephone.com*.

Polycom. (n.d.). Retrieved July 20, 2008, from *www.polycom.com/index2.html*.

Skype. (n.d.). Retrieved July 20, 2008, from *www.skype.com*.

TelSpan. (n.d.). Retrieved July 20, 2008, from *www.telspan.com*.

Test your Internet connection speed. (n.d.). Speakeasy, Inc. Retrieved July 20, 2008, from *www.speakeasy.net/ speedtest/*.

The Webcast Academy. (n.d.). Retrieved July 20, 2008, from *www.webcastacademy.net/About_Webcast_Academy*.

Video webcast center. (n.d.). U.S. Food and Drug Administration. Retrieved July 20, 2008, from *www. accessdata.fda.gov/psn/viewbroadcasts.cfm*.

Webex. (n.d.). Retrieved July 20, 2008, from *www.webex.com*.

New Technology in Nursing Staff Development

Web-based training and online databases

LEARNING OBJECTIVES

After reading this chapter, the participant will be able to:

- List four of the most common types of Web-based communication

- Discuss copyright considerations in relation to Web-based training

Remember the television show "The Wonderful World of Disney"? Well, this chapter is all about "The Wonderful World of Web." For educators who enjoy distributed education, the Web is a wonderful, wonderful thing. It's like having a new jigsaw puzzle—you know what the ultimate goal is because you can see the picture on the box, but how you choose to approach the solution is uniquely you. Everything you have or will read about in this book, with the possible exception of simulation, can be used with Web-based teaching and training. It's like your favorite smorgasbord where you can pick and choose, mix and match, return for seconds, and have dessert, too.

The World Wide Web (also called the Web or WWW) was created in the early 1990s, and Web-based education began being used in the mid- to late-90s. This is not to say that educators didn't use the Web before that time, but the first Web-based offerings took the form of simple lists of links, evolving into static pages of text with perhaps an image or two added for visual appeal. These simple beginnings gave Web-based learning a bad reputation as being nothing more than an online book, one that learners generally printed in order to read at their convenience while off-line. For some individuals, that's where the Web stayed, but it's so much more than that. If you're a skeptic, perhaps we can convince you that it's a magical, wonderful World Wide Web out there. Cue the theme music.

Technical details

Elements presented via the Web—text, images, podcasts, audio, video, or interactive learning activities—are served (delivered after a request is received) from a Web server. The request is made with a click of the mouse on a Web page via a Web browser. There are many, many Web browsers, but only two consistently retain market dominance: Firefox and Internet Explorer. Although their components and commands are arranged differently or called by slightly different names, they have the same basic functionality.

Web pages are most often created through markup languages called HTML (HyperText Markup Language) or XML (eXtensible Markup Language). HTML is the original language of the Web; XML is the current language, although HTML continues to be accepted widely by browsers, created by users, and used by millions of Web pages. How the markup languages work and the details of how to create Web documents are described in numerous books and online resources, so we won't attempt to teach you that here. Nevertheless, you need some background on how they work.

A standard text document has codes added to it. These codes are instructions that specify how the text on the page is supposed to look—formatting and layout, for example. Codes also may be instructions on how to retrieve and display additional elements, such as images, other pages, and audio and video files, or how to access other resources such as online databases.

Now, you may be thinking, "I don't want to know how to do all of that!" That's one of the beauties of the Web; you don't have to (although there are many who believe that a fundamental understanding of how Web documents are created will help you to understand the possibilities and to unravel mysteries when pages don't display the way you intended). There are many WYSIWYG (What-You-See-Is-What-You-Get) editors available, both commercial and free. Although they each offer the same basic functionality, there are differences in ease of use, interface, and robustness, in addition to cost. If you are creating Web documents for your institution or that need to work with Web content created by and for your institution, check

 New Technology in Nursing Staff Development

with your network staff to see what product is most compatible with your technologies. Some Web page applications include:

- Adobe Dreamweaver (*www.adobe.com*)

- Microsoft FrontPage (which is no longer being developed by Microsoft) (*http://office. microsoft.com/frontpage*)

- Nvu (*http://nvudev.com*)

- Amaya (*www.w3.org/Amaya*)

Learning management systems

As mentioned above, all documents on the Web are served from a Web server. Of special interest to educators are learning management systems (LMSs). An LMS is a special software family that is installed on a Web server. Blackboard (*www.blackboard.com*), WebCT (*www. webct.com*) (which now has been purchased by Blackboard), ANGEL (*www.angellearning.com*), Moodle (*http://moodle.org*), and SAKAI (*http://sakaiproject.org*) are currently available mainstream LMSs.

An LMS creates the structure for teaching and learning online. It may provide tools such as student enrollment, online communication, collaboration, and assessment. It's not that any or all of those functions can't be developed or added to stand-alone Web sites, but an LMS provides a comprehensive package with a standard set of tools and a common interface.

Let's use this example to illustrate: A good lumberyard contains all of the supplies necessary for you to build and decorate your own home. You can even request instructions on how to get started—all you need to do is create the plan, purchase all of the components, put them together in the correct way and, voilá!, you have a house. (Not necessarily something you want to do, or have the expertise or time to do, but it is possible.) On the other hand, you could purchase the services of an architect who will draw up the plans for you according to your needs and desires, a general contractor who will oversee the project on your behalf and hire the crew who is experienced in building houses, and an interior designer to help you choose interesting décor and color palettes. All you need to do is work within the guidelines that your selected experts provide and approve or disapprove plans in order to create your dream home.

Granted, this example is very simplistic, but it demonstrates the difference between creating pages, developing resources, and knowing how to hook them all together to create a Web-based course, versus having a system in place where others have created the structure that allows you to plug in the components you desire in order to achieve the result you need. It's not that the latter is necessarily simple or without effort, but plugging in pieces is definitely easier than nailing two-by-fours or cutting down timber.

Good LMSs allow educators to:

- Upload documents

- Manage content

- Structure communication through mail, threaded discussion forums, chat, and announcements

- Create and maintain calendars or schedules

- Administer courses including enrollment, learners' and educators' roles, and course environments

- Assess and evaluate

- Incorporate additional tools needed to meet learning outcomes

Additional, optional components include the capability for the educator to:

- Adjust course content on the fly

- Add/delete/organize tools

- Create new functionality personalized to the educator, course goals, and/or learners

- Integrate seamlessly with other available teaching and learning tools and environments

- Provide historical tracking of changes

- Create SCORM-compliant content (SCORM is an industry standard that allows a package to be created of a course that is usable by other systems, rather than being usable only by other installations of the same LMS)

Web content

Unlike a book, which a reader most often starts at the beginning and proceeds through the chapters consecutively, the Web encourages readers to start wherever they need or want to, and to navigate through the content in whatever ways best meet their learning needs. Educators need to keep this in mind as they develop content and organize it. The Web is a hypertext environment, which means that by clicking a link, the learner can move to another part of the course or to a new resource that you've created, or to another Web site altogether. Where a learner starts is not necessarily where you, the educator, expected or planned for the starting point to be.

Audience analysis

As an educator, you should determine who exactly your audience is and build a learning segment (be it a course, a module, or a short tutorial) for that audience. This is not to say that branches along the primary trunk of the course shouldn't exist. That's the beauty of the Web: branches can and should exist. For example, assume that you are developing a learning module for the novice emergency room nurse. This nurse may have several years of nursing experience behind him or her but may wish to move into this new area of nursing. This foundational assessment of your audience allows you to structure your content so that you don't need to start at the definitions and explanations that would be necessary for a new nursing graduate. Once you identify the primary path, you can easily incorporate branches in which you provide supplemental or enhancement content or activities for the nurse who may have gained some emergency care nursing knowledge throughout the years or for the learner who wants to go the extra mile. You also can provide branches that contain remediation content and activities for those instances in which you believe that learners might need a boost or reminder.

Organizing content

Consistency is a hallmark in Web-based training and education. Learners who have been provided with an introduction to the course should be able to enter any component of it and know where they are in relation to the rest of the course and how to find necessary content. Consider a print textbook. Books usually have a front and back cover, publication information in the front, a table of contents, an introduction, a brief author biography, the chapters, and sometimes an index. You don't have to learn how to read that particular book; you can simply begin. In other words, a learner should not have to learn how to learn within each section—the learner should be able to dive in and begin learning the content. The way that an educator can support this process is through a consistent organization of content.

How you elect to organize your content is based on your own preferences and teaching style, as well as the anticipated learning styles of the learners. If you have access to an instructional designer, this knowledge expert can provide guidance and direction in these tasks. Here are some guidelines:

- Each module should begin with an overview. It is not sufficient to have only a course overview provided in the syllabus or a welcome sheet. Remember that learners access Web content via different channels. A learner may not have started by reading the syllabus as you intended. Overviews to each module or unit should be formatted consistently and displayed so that learners can quickly jump into learning the content within that section.

- Each module should contain learning objectives and components that are organized consistently. You may decide that each module should contain a brief list of terms and definitions pertinent to that content, provide a list of required and recommended learning activities, and identify required and supplemental readings for that module. Use whatever strategy you decide will best enable the learner to reach the learning outcomes.

- The content should be structured in a logical manner that allows learners to navigate directly to needed content. The general rule of thumb in structuring Web content is a funnel, allowing learners to drill down from broad topics, down to focused topics, and finally to specific details.

Here are some examples of how to structure content:

- A Web-based seminar to teach practicing nurses about nurse practitioner (NP) roles might be organized first by topic (e.g., clinical reasoning, dermatology, microscope use, musculoskeletal, head/eyes/ears/nose/throat), since there would be information on each topic that is needed by all NPs, and then by role (e.g., women's health NP, pediatric NP, acute care NP, family NP, adult NP, and neonatal NP), since the broad topic would drill down into details uniquely required by the individual NP roles.

- A course to train practicing nurses in critical care nursing might be organized first by audience (e.g., adult, pediatric, and neonatal), then by body system (e.g., respiratory, cardio-vascular, gastrointestinal, neurology), and then it might drill down to specific etiologies.

 New Technology in Nursing Staff Development

- A module for new nursing staff educators might be organized into the key functions of the role (e.g., managing a clinical day, planning learning activities, and evaluating learning), which would drill down to specific tasks within those functions.

In each of these examples, learners are free to proceed through the course or module sequentially or randomly based on their needs. You may be wondering how to ensure that fundamental learning occurs before jumping into new concepts, since we know that new knowledge is built on existing knowledge. There are several strategies that you might employ, either singularly or in combination.

In the course introduction, you might explain that while learners are free to navigate through the content as they desire, communication and assignments will cover specific content according to the posted schedule and that the learners are responsible for qualitative contributions during the specified time period.

You might elect to hyperlink key concepts in the content to the first in-depth explanation of that concept. Although this approach will help learners who find that they need that background, there are two distinct disadvantages to weigh:

1. When you later edit your course, you will need to take particular care that you check each hyperlink to ensure that you don't inadvertently leave a link that doesn't go to its intended destination

2. You risk learners going off on a learning tangent and not returning to the section from whence they came (although there are some who would say that learning is learning, and that this isn't a disadvantage)

A third strategy is to guide learners through the course by the way you create the linking. For example, there may be components of the course where you feel that it is absolutely critical that the content be traversed in a specific way. In these sections, you might encourage the learner to read through the content sequentially by not building any hyperlinked content. In other sections of the course, however, you might build several different navigation schemas to allow the learners to learn in the directions that they choose.

Developing content

Many educators are well versed in writing for publication and may have learned certain general writing rules. As you may have noticed from this book, the tone and voice are decidedly informal—but not unprofessional—when compared to a scholarly research article. Writing for the Web is much the same. Content is usually written in the first person, it is more informal than scholarly writing, and sentences, paragraphs, and modules are short and easy to scan.

This scan-ability factor is a goal in writing for the Web. Jakob Neilson, a recognized authority on Web usability since the Web's inception, documented as long ago as 1997 research showing that 79% of Web users scanned pages rather than reading them word for word. As the pace of most of our lives has continued to quicken in the ensuing years, and as younger learners are more apt to be accustomed to texting, e-mailing, and other quick forms of communication, this statistic is sure to have even greater ramifications.

Web pages contain three distinct areas of "real estate:" white space, black space, and gray space. White space includes the gaps—margins, vertical spacing, and spacing around tables, images, and charts. Black space includes the densest areas: images. Gray space encompasses the text and other elements on a page. When developing Web documents, leave sufficient white space so that important elements stand out and catch the reader's attention as he or she scans a page.

One way to ensure scan-ability is to recognize that headings play a very important role in Web page development and that the words you use must pack a lot of punch to encourage learners to read sections in the text. It also means that white space is an important consideration in Web development.

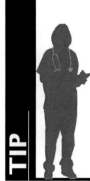

TIP

After you have developed a Web page, print it out and have someone several feet away from you hold it up (or you can squint at it as you hold it). Your eyes should easily discern margins, locations of images, beginnings of new sections, etc. If they do so, then you know you have sufficient white space. When testing multiple pages in this manner, your eyes should determine the patterns of where new sections begin and be able to anticipate how the content is structured. Don't add space just for the sake of adding space, though. Be consistent and thoughtful.

New Technology in Nursing Staff Development

To aid scan-ability, Web developers should consider how to format content on a Web page.

- If you choose to bold many words (because we all know that everything educators write is important), then none of the bolded text retains any emphasis (think of the boy who cried wolf—one cry attracted attention; multiple cries simply caused him to be ignored).

- If you create headings in many different colors or emphasize words and phrases with different colors throughout the content, then the consistency that readers depend upon is lost. Therefore, ensure that the same colors are used consistently and retain the same meaning throughout the content.

- Place images carefully. In Western cultures, pages are read from top to bottom and from left to right. If you place an image on the left and the text flows to the right, the image assumes the most importance. If you place the image on the right and allow the text to wrap around the left then the text assumes the most importance.

- If you change the alignment of key components, you discourage a reader's ability to scan for comprehension.

Placement and alignment of page components can enhance or detract from a learner's ability to scan the page for important elements. The Web Style Guide (found at *www.webstyleguide.com*) has an excellent article on this topic. It goes into great detail about why it's important to left-align text and headings in Web pages, and it includes visual aids to illustrate these important concepts.

Three text elements are always present on a Web page: text, hyperlinks, and visited hyperlinks. Text is, well, text. Hyperlinks are words and phrases on which an individual can click in order to access something different. Visited hyperlinks are links that a person has already clicked. By default, text is black, hyperlinks are blue, and visited hyperlinks are purple. It's not necessary that you keep the default colors, but it is important that these three text elements are colored uniquely and complementarily. A learner's ability to scan a page and to see at a glance where the text is, where the hyperlinks are, and which hyperlinks have already been visited greatly enhances working on the Web.

The color wheel that can be found on this book's accompanying CD can be used as a guide in color selection. When you read through this section, note that there is a difference between human applications of colors (think crayons) and the use of colors in printing or computing. In printing, primary colors are those that are not combined with any other color to get the resulting color. For example, magenta, yellow, and cyan (those three colors shown in the outer ring) are simply the colors they are. When working with computer printers, you may have seen the designation CMYK—these stand for cyan, magenta, yellow, and black. These are the basic, primary colors that serve as the foundation for all other colors. When adjacent pairs of primary colors are blended, secondary colors, shown in the inner ring, are formed. For example, magenta and cyan blend to form blue. Yellow and cyan blend to form green, and so on. For good contrast, choose pairs of primary colors. For complementary colors, select a primary color and the secondary color that falls opposite it on the color wheel (cyan and red; yellow and blue; magenta and green).

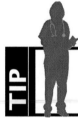

TIP Avoid red-green color combinations due to the high percentage of individuals (particularly males) who have a red-green color deficiency.

Web-based communication

We've spent considerable time talking about Web pages; however, one of the most important contributions to education that Web-based learning offers is communication. The Web is full of ways for communication to occur. This section discusses four of the most common and their advantages and disadvantages: announcements, mail, chat, and discussion forums.

Announcements

Educators use announcements, which include time-sensitive information, to provide one-way information to the learners. They generally should take the form of headlines—not excessive detail, but enough detail to encourage further delving into the information if needed. An LMS should allow educators to add start and stop dates to announcements so that they can specify the number of days that an announcement should run. The capability to specify start dates allows educators to preload announcements.

New Technology in Nursing Staff Development

For example, assume that you know you will be attending a World's Best Online Web Instructor conference in the fall and that you're also scheduled to teach a specific ongoing class in the fall. You've made arrangements for a guest lecturer to monitor communications and interact with the learners in your absence. As you prepare your upcoming clinical education, you can add an announcement, reminding the learners of the dates you will be out of town. Then, on the date you are first due to be absent, you can schedule an announcement introducing the guest lecturer and providing links to an introduction and details of any assignments that are due while you're gone. On the specified date, each announcement can automatically "drop off" without the need for you to set a reminder for yourself to remove them.

Mail

Many educators and learners have electronic mail (e-mail) and use it both professionally and personally, so the concept of e-mail isn't unfamiliar. Using it in relation to educational work may be, however. Many LMSs have built-in mail functionality. Although some systems allow you to use regular e-mail, others have a self-contained e-mail system that works only within the confines of a specific educational course. There are both advantages and disadvantages to this system. Some people receive a great deal of e-mail daily and appreciate knowing that education-related mail isn't interspersed with personal and professional mail. For these individuals, knowing that they can rely on mail pertaining to particular training to remain in that mail folder helps them to stay organized. The flipside of the coin are those who do not want to go to multiple systems to check mail and want all mail, regardless of its origin, to be delivered to regular e-mail accounts.

In a Web-based educational course, mail can be used most effectively in one-to-many or one-to-one correspondence. By design, it is not particularly effective at encouraging deep-level conversations among groups of participants. E-mail is an asynchronous mode of communication, meaning that participants do not have to be online at the same time and that sending and receiving messages may be time-delayed and depend upon when a user logs on. Advantages of Web-based mail include the following:

- Users are not required to be online at a particular time

- Responses can be developed thoroughly and reviewed before being sent

- Communication can be spell-checked and contain at least minimal formatting (depending on the system)

- Messages can be private (sent to a single individual) or public (sent to the entire group)

Disadvantages of e-mail include:

- Delayed response times result from users logging on at different times. This can lead to "strung out" conversations that are difficult to conclude successfully.

- Lack of robust formatting capabilities makes it difficult to submit assignments

Chat

Chat is a real-time, synchronous, mode of communication. For the conversation to occur, participants must be online at the same time and accessing the same chat room. Chats can be private if the system allows it, but they are primarily public to anyone who happens to be in the chat room at the same time. Some systems provide for a chat, or a particular chat room, to be archived for later access.

For chats to be most effective, there should be ten or fewer participants; above that number, conversations become disjointed and race along more quickly than most participants can process. Chats favor fast typists and quick thinkers. Those who ponder carefully or who are slower typists are left behind as the conversation surges ahead without them.

Teaching strategies that effectively use chat include:

- Online office hours

- Brainstorming sessions

- Small group work

- Question-and-answer sessions

Discussion forums

Discussion forums, also called threaded discussion or bulletin boards, are another form of asynchronous communication. Participants do not have to be online at the same time or active simultaneously in the forum in order to communicate. Although some systems allow a forum to be access restricted to a particular group or individual, they are generally accessible to any participant of the course.

Forums are referred to as threaded because it is easy to see strands of conversation. For example, an educator may post a discussion question regarding the case study being studied in that unit. A learner will post a reply to that initial posting, beginning a thread of a conversation. Subsequent posts may either be replies to the educator's initial posting or replies to other reply postings.

Threading is one of the most important skills in effectively communicating in discussion forums. Assume that a group of nursing students are conducting a post-clinical debriefing in a discussion forum. Each student will post a new thread to indicate that she or he is discussing the cases presented during the shift. Other students, the educator, and perhaps the preceptors will post replies to various postings adding clarifying information, insights gained, or posing questions; each of these postings will be indented in a cascade that shows the relationship to the original posting. Now assume that Student M wants to ask a question regarding Student B's case and doesn't understand threading. Instead of posting in Student B's thread, Student M posts a new message that simply reads, "I don't understand how that could have happened and what the impact would be on the patient. Can you explain further?" How will any of the participants know which case this question pertains to?

Advantages of forums include the ability to:

- Compose responses thoughtfully and check spelling and grammar

- Request or provide additional information

- Alleviate the effect of time zone differences

- Allow communication to occur at times convenient to participants

Discussion forums are the backbone of most Web-based teaching and training due to their flexibility and versatility. Here are some teaching and learning strategies for you to consider when developing forums:

- **Round Robins.** This strategy encourages learners to post early. To respond to a scenario or question, no poster can replicate what a previous post said. Not only does this rule encourage learners to post early so that "all of the good answers" aren't used, it causes learners to read each others' postings in order to know what was previously posted.

- **Debates.** This strategy is perhaps one of the most flexible because educators can tweak it however they desire. Here's one option: Learners are randomly assigned to either the pro or con position. A scenario is developed and posted by the educator. In the specified time period, the debaters must develop their positions, including references and drawing in research as applicable, in their posts. Because a learner's personal position may not be the position to which she/he is assigned, it causes the development of sound logic and promotes research in order to support the assigned position.

- **Group exercises.** In group assignments, the group must discuss and develop their response to the posed assignment. One member of the group takes on the responsibility of group recorder and another of group poster. Other roles are developed as needed. When consensus has been reached, the group prepares their formal response, and the poster submits on behalf of the group. Not only does this strategy promote team work, consensus building, and writing skills, it also cuts down the number of postings that the educator must read, since there is only a single post from each group.

- **Online journals.** In this strategy, your LMS must support private forums. Learners must be able to be assured that no one other than the educator will be privy to their personal thoughts and reflections.

- **Assignment submission.** Traditionally, assignments are prepared by a learner and submitted only to the educator. In this strategy, all learner work is posted to a public forum that is accessible to other participants. One educator's experience with this strategy is that learners first complain and are fearful of this openness, but by the end of the course, they praise the amount of learning that occurred. Except for grading comments, all educator comments regarding a learner's work are posted publicly. This open exchange allows learners to learn from one another and from the educator. It helps slower learners by providing guidance and direction, and it encourages high-achieving learners to assume leadership roles by providing opportunities for them to help other learners.

Other Web-based communication

Briefly, here are some other Web strategies and communication tools that educators are apt to see discussed and may wish to explore:

New Technology in Nursing Staff Development

- **Wikis:** Online collaborative tools. The most widely recognized wiki is Wikipedia (*www.wikipedia.org*). This collaborative strategy allows learners to add, delete, and edit a Web-based document collaboratively. Using a simple coding schema, users can format a document and add links to additional resources to build a rich resource. Most wikis are self-policed—and, indeed, this is one of the cornerstones of this strategy—meaning that there is no moderator through which content must pass, but the users themselves learn, build, and verify content. To see how wikis are being used in education, look at Educational Wikis (*http://educationalwikis.wikispaces.com*). As an educational strategy, wikis encourage collaboration to produce a written product.

- **Blogs (weB-LOGS):** An online journal. Blogs are usually created by individuals and may be a stream-of-consciousness series of postings or dedicated to a particular topic. Content may include text, images, audio/video, or links to other sites. Will Richardson, who developed Weblogg-ed (the Read/Write Web), at *http://weblogg-ed.com*, may be one of the most well-known educators involved in blogging, wikis, podcasting, and other Web tools.

- **Texting:** Many adults have been a bit slow to jump on the text messaging bandwagon, considering it a tool for teens and those of nimble thumbs. However, educational texting has begun to receive considerable press recently. In the article, "Using text messaging to support administrative communication in higher education," found in the journal *Active Learning for Higher Education*, author Laura Naismith (2007) reports that "tutors reported changes in behavior that were directly attributable to the use of text messaging." Texting is a strategy that should remain on educator's horizon as time goes on.

Teaching and learning strategies

Traditionally, Web-based teaching and training has been heavily focused in two primary areas: content and communication. With changes in technology—faster and more affordable connections, better graphics, more robust computing power—many other strategies are available to educators. Let's take a brief look at a few of the additional teaching strategies that educators might consider:

- **Web-based simulation.** Simulation is a way to learn in a non threatening, cost-effective, safe manner. Chapter 5 discusses simulation. But educators can also consider Web-based simulation. Drag-and-drop simulations allow learners to use a computer mouse to simulate actions. For example, a drag-and-drop exercise might allow a learner to correctly sequence and place EKG sensors and cables on a patient; a simulated stethoscope allows a learner to identify breath sounds; or virtual slides educate a learner on pathology. For a starter list of Web sites, visit Web by Design's Active Learning resources at *www.iupui.edu/~webtrain/active_learning.html*.

- **Webquests.** This inquiry-oriented strategy can be used by educators with individual learners or groups of learners. Learners are provided with a topic, a task, and usually a beginning list of resources. The learning occurs as the questors work through the process of arriving at a successful conclusion of the specified task.

- **Guest experts.** The Internet has greatly shrunk our universe. Through the power of the Web, educators can invite experts to visit their classrooms virtually and to interact with learners. One strategy is to invite an expert to log in to the online classroom for a short, specified period of time. Learners and expert interact through chats and/or discussion forums.

- **Problem-based learning (PBL).** In PBL, learners are presented with an ill-defined case or scenario—in other words, a real-world problem—and as they work through the problem, additional information is revealed. This strategy promotes critical thinking and reflection and can be used with all levels of learners from novice to expert.

- **Presentations.** Do you think that PowerPoint needs to be presented live in a classroom? Think again. Learners can develop a presentation and publish it on a class Web site or in an online classroom.

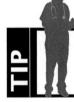

TIP

When PowerPoint is coupled with other technologies, such as chats, forums, or podcasts, the learner can share the presentation virtually.

Web 2.0

Web 2.0 is the term being used to describe the "next wave" in the Web. It is based on creativity and interactivity. Wikis and blogs both fall into the Web 2.0 domain. Tim O'Reilly of O'Reilly Media also categorizes Skype and Flickr, an online photo and video sharing service, among Web 2.0 technologies.

New Technology in Nursing Staff Development

Another important genre in Web 2.0 is social networking services such as MySpace and Facebook, both of which were once relegated to the world of teens and twentysomethings but now are becoming standards in education and business. An advanced form of social network is virtual worlds such as Second Life, through which learners are personified through their chosen avatars (the computer's image representation of the student). This environment is not only virtual and collaborative but also has a strong simulation component, since participants can interact and perform in ways that might be unavailable, risky, or costly in the real world.

Searching the Web effectively

Since we've spent considerable time discussing Web pages and teaching technologies, let's spend some time discussing how educators can find resources that already exist and can be incorporated into Web-based courses. Metamend, a search engine marketing company, estimates that there are more than 17 billion publicly accessible Web pages in existence. Is it any wonder, then, that we often have difficulty finding accurate, timely, and evidence-based information on the Web?

There are many resources published to help educators search more effectively. One particularly effective method is the STAIR method:

- State your question to eliminate jargon

- Tools (determine the best ones to use to achieve your objective)

- Approach (understand how the tool works best)

- Implement your search

- Refine search until you receive satisfactory results

Prior to using the STAIR method (shown in Figure 3.1) to begin a search, educators may want to complete a guide that will help them analyze their search criteria. In 2004, Joseph Barker of the University of California, Berkeley Teaching Library developed a topic worksheet (find it at *www.lib.berkeley.edu/TeachingLib/Guides/Internet/form.pdf*) that guides you through a pre-searching analysis. You can print and complete this document so that when you do begin to conduct your online searches, your time will be more efficient and your search more effective.

FIGURE
3.1

The STAIR method

State your question to eliminate jargon

Some people perform Web searches by typing a word or two into the location/address area of the browser then clicking the Go or Google button to start the search. Others go to a search site and type words into the keywords box. The result in either of these types of searches is generally millions of hits—sites that possibly meet your specified criteria—many of which have nothing to do with the information you are seeking. For example, if you type CHF into the Google search tool because you want information on congestive heart failure, you will receive more than 10 million hits. Topics will include the consumers' health forum, the Canadian Hunger Foundation, Cosgrove Hall Films, and congestive heart failure. To search more effectively, use the words "congestive heart failure" rather than using the jargon "CHF".

Tools (determine the best ones to use to achieve your objective)

The term "search engine" is used as a generic descriptor for those tools that let us search for files on the Web. In reality, there are several different types of search tools available on the Web. Each of them looks at different Web sites in different ways; therefore, the results you get when using the tools may vary considerably:

- Search engine: A database of publicly accessible Web sites. This automated process programmatically adds each page it locates to an index. When a search is conducted using a search engine, the engine retrieves a listing from its database of each Web site containing the specified keyword(s). Because there are millions of pages on the Web, a search engine cannot be completely accurate and might, in fact, be greatly out-of-date. There also will be pages that are not added to the index because some systems are programmed to locate sites only by following links, which would mean that a page containing no links would not be indexed. Some Web pages have instructions added to them requiring the page to remain unindexed. Two-well known search engines are Google (*www.google.com*) and Ask (*www.ask.com*).

- Meta search engine: A clearinghouse search engine. It sends the keyword(s) to several different search engine databases simultaneously. The returned list is the same list you would have received if you had visited each of the search engine sites individually and performed the search multiple times. Each meta search engine does not search the same set of databases; if you want the best results, conduct searches using different meta search engines so that you are accessing a variety of engines. Two popular meta search engines are Dogpile (*www.dogpile.com/*) and AllinOne (*www.searchallinone.com/*).

New Technology in Nursing Staff Development

FIGURE
3.1

The STAIR method (cont.)

- **Subject directories:** Human-generated and organized systems. Main categories are developed and then divided and subdivided so that searchers drill down to get to requested information. Because they are human generated, subject directories generally do not contain as many resources as do search engines. Two commonly used subject directories are About (*www. about.com*) and Yahoo (*http://dir.yahoo.com*).

- **Library gateways:** Human generated and maintained; more likely than most general search engines to be organized, researched, and maintained by specialists—in this case, librarians. These gateways link to specific databases that are generally more reliable sources of resources than subject directories. They are commonly academically or research oriented. Two popular library gateways are the Librarians' Internet Index (*http://lii.org/*) and LibWeb (*http://lists. webjunction.org/libweb/*).

- **Subject-specific databases:** Some of the previously discussed tools, such as Yahoo, can be defined as portals—a door that opens to a wide array of topics, often very broad but not very deep. Subject-specific databases are resources known as vortals—a vertical portal—that opens to a narrow, yet deep, array of information on a specific topic or type of topics. WebMD (*www.webmd.com*) is a popular subject-specific database for obtaining health-related information, and ERIC (*www.eric.ed.gov*) provides access to millions of bibliographic records of journal articles and other education-related materials.

CINAHL Information Systems and Medline are two subject-specific databases of interest to nursing. CINAHL's database contains nursing and allied health literature. To help users learn how to access and search CINAHL effectively, the University of Florida Health Science Center Libraries in Gainsville has published an online tutorial that may be accessed at *www.citt.ufl.edu/portfolio/cinahl/*.

MEDLINE contains resources for the life sciences and biomedical fields. MEDLINE is searched using medical subject headings (MeSH) rather than keywords. The Bibliographic Services Division of the National Library of Medicine (*www.nlm.nih.gov/bsd/disted/video/windows/*) has created many tools that will help you search MEDLINE effectively, including a video on the MeSH vocabulary.

FIGURE 3.1

The STAIR method (cont.)

Approach (understand how the tool works best)

Effective search strategies avoid the use of jargon, choose the right tool, and specify exactly what you're seeking. A multiword keyword phrase generates a listing of every document that has any one, but not necessarily all, of the keywords. For example, assume that you want information on infusion nursing. If you search using that keyword phrase in Google, it will return a listing of more than 1.2 million hits, with only a relatively small number actually pertaining to infusion nursing. Some of the list will be information about infusion, but most of the sites will be information about nursing. Obviously, that strategy isn't precise enough.

To indicate that you want information on the topic infusion nursing, place the phrase in quotations: "infusion nursing." Doing so tells the search tool to search for that specific phrase and return only those documents that contain the entire phrase. When you use Google and search for the keyword phrase, it decreases the number of hits to a little more than 41,000—still an impressive number, but not nearly as intimidating (or misleading) as more than 1.2 million!

Searchers also use wildcards, a specific character that substitutes for one or more unspecified or unknown characters. The asterisk is the most common wildcard. For example, to search for information on anesthesia, anesthesiology, anesthetists, and anesthesiologists, use the search term anesth* in order to receive a list containing all those variants.

Implement your search and refine search until you receive satisfactory results

The final two steps in the STAIR are to 1) implement the search and 2) refine the search until you receive satisfactory results. After you have avoided using jargon, chosen the right tools, and learned how the tool best functions, you are ready to implement your search. Just as conducting research in a library doesn't result in the perfect resource the first time, so it is with Web searching. Remember: to get the best results, you have to explore, test, and refine your search.

Source: Andrew Harris. Indiana University School of Nursing. Used with permission.

Copyright considerations

Web-based training and teaching provides educators opportunities to marry a variety of learning tools and strategies in order to help learners achieve the learning outcomes. As anyone who is comfortable surfing the Web knows, it is easy to find numerous resources including articles and images to use in Web classrooms. With these resources, though, comes the responsibility of using them legally and professionally.

Nearly everything that is created and stored in a fixed medium is copyrighted by the author/creator/developer (this doesn't address work for hire and other exceptions, which is beyond what we can cover here). For educators, this means that the image you find using Google's image search (and that is the exact visual you need in your lesson) is copyrighted. Just because it is easy for you to "save as" and use the image doesn't mean that you have permission to do so. Fortunately, there are many resources on the Web that are created by and for educational uses. Educators need to look for and read Web sites for acceptable use statements (often listed along with copyright information).

Another area besides graphics that cause educators frustration is works that they themselves have created. Authors must realize that most journals own the copyright of published articles. This means that even if you wrote the article on "Ideal techniques for conducting in-home interviews of the elderly," you need to check the statement you signed with the publisher of that work. Unless you retained the specific rights to republish that work, you need to obtain the publisher's permission before including it as a resource in your Web-based course.

There are exceptions to obtaining permissions, and they fall under the copyright law's Fair Use Exception. This provision provides educators the opportunity to use copyrighted works without obtaining permission. The Copyright Advisory Office of Columbia University Libraries/Information Services Web site has graciously provided permission for educators to use the Fair Use Checklist (*www.copyright.columbia.edu/fair-use-checklist*). This easy-to-use form allows educators to answer a series of questions and place checkmarks against answers in one of two columns, Favoring Fair Use and Opposing Fair Use. After answering all the questions, the educator counts up the checkmarks in each column, and the column with the most checkmarks determines whether the use of the material leans toward fair use. If, when finished, the scales are tipped toward fair use, then no permission is needed. Educators are encouraged to complete and store a checklist for each copyrighted work that they wish to use in Web-based course so that if questions ever arise, they can demonstrate good-faith effort to comply with copyright law.

If the checklist does not indicate fair use, then seek permission from the copyright holder. Sample permission letters are included with the chapter on podcasting and audio/visual and are also included on Columbia's Web site. Make sure that your requests for permission are detailed requests outlining your purpose and intent.

Financial considerations

With the exception of Web servers and learning management systems (LMS), many of the tools that we've discussed in this chapter are freely available on the World Wide Web. Others are available for nominal costs.

If you are unable to locate the perfect resource to use in your online course or learning segment, consider hiring a university's new media or graphic design student to work on your project. These students are learning their skills and looking to build portfolios of work they have developed. They are generally creative, have access to expensive software and the knowledge of skilled faculty professionals, and work inexpensively—a win-win situation!

Evaluating your options

Web-based resources open additional opportunities for educators and learners alike. As we've demonstrated in this chapter, online databases can be a great asset to the staff educator and nursing faculty. Most publishers and many professional organizations provide online resources for nurses and nursing organizations. When evaluating whether or not Web-based learning is right for you, check with your local schools of nursing, medicine, and allied health, as well as with professional organizations, to see whether you are able to negotiate opportunities for your staff to access online resources.

Deciding on the right technology

To succeed in today's world of technology, we all have to work smarter, not harder. And quite often that means that we must search for resources and not always think that we need to start from scratch each time. Consider the following questions when deciding whether Web-based learning is right for you:

- **Rather than jumping full stream into Web-based learning, could you consider blended learning?** Blended learning, which is discussed in an upcoming chapter, allows you to use the best of the face-to-face and online worlds. Not only will this allow educators to choose from a broader variety of training and educational options, but it keeps things interesting for learners and educators alike. Use Web-based learning for those areas that need consistency and are fundamental and the face-to-face time for those things that are best accomplished in your own institution one-to-one or in small groups.

- **Are you able to provide adequate support and initial training to your learners?** If you are considering Web-based training, it is important that your students are provided with this preparation. Consider requesting that learners take online "Am I ready for online learning?" assessments to identify their understanding of Web-based learning, identify areas where they are likely to need additional support, and to identify whether they have adequate computing resources to make the training venue feasible.

Justifying your resources

For staff educators, Web-based learning doesn't always have to mean purchasing an LMS and putting all offerings into this format. It is simply another viable alternative to meeting the needs of learners. This is an essential point when justifying Web-based training.

If your facility is new to this venue, consider partnering with other organizations. For example, many schools of nursing offer continuing education in Web-based formats. It may be that organizations can negotiate to allow groups of nurses access to already-created Web offerings at a discount. Not only would this result in a cost savings since your organization doesn't have to develop these offerings, but you're saving money over the costs of individual enrollment fees and the nurses are earning contact hours toward professional development requirements. for example, some staff educators have found that they can send new preceptors through a nursing school's online preceptor program, freeing up their face-to-face classroom time for institution-specific needs.

Obtaining administrative buy-in

For administrators, it is important that you are able to demonstrate that it's not necessary for them to throw their entire educational department out the door in order to have learners participate in Web-based learning. Start slow and build successes. Don't reinvent the wheel. If there are resources in place at other institutions and organizations, negotiate, partner, and team up so that everyone walks away in a win-win situation.

In addition, many professional journals and organizations are requiring authors, editors, and reviewers to use online interfaces. These changes indicate that online is here to stay and educators, nurses, and other professionals need to become at least somewhat comfortable in these environments. Emphasize this point to your administrators as you attempt to gain their buy-in and support.

Obtaining staff buy-in

For learners, understanding Web-based learning is the most important facet of success in this type of education. If learners believe that they are going to learn more in less time, that it is less demanding, that they can skip corners and go right to the test, then it is likely that they will be frustrated in online learning. When learners need to see the people they are interacting with and thrive in environments where they are isolated from other demands of life by the rooms of the classroom, then they may find that Web-based learning is not for them.

Educators need to understand the unique characteristics of their learners and to help them build a strong foundation for success as the attempt to gain their buy-in for this new technology. Only then can Web-based learning be a viable option for an institution.

Conclusion

Web-based teaching and learning isn't the easy path around the rigors of academia. It is hard work, but with careful planning, the assistance of experts such as instructional designers and online learning experts, and time to become comfortable with the environment, it is a rich and rewarding environment for the educator and learner.

References

About. (n.d.). Retrieved July 22, 2008, from *http://www.about.com*.

A little history of the World Wide Web. (2006, June 13). World Wide Web Consortium. Retrieved July 20, 2008 from *http://www.w3.org/History.html*.

All-In-One. (n.d.). Retrieved July 22, 2008, from *http://www.searchallinone.com*.

Amaya. (n.d.). World Wide Consortium. Retrieved July 20, 2008, from *http://www.w3.org/Amaya/Amaya.html*.

ANGEL. (n.d.). Retrieved July 20, 2008, from *http://www.angellearning.com*.

Ask. (n.d.). Retrieved July 22, 2008, from *http://www.ask.com*.

Barker, J. (2004). Topic worksheet. Retrieved July 22, 2008, from the Teaching Library, University of California, Berkeley Web site: *http://www.lib.berkeley.edu/TeachingLib/Guides/Internet/form.pdf*.

Blackboard. (n.d.). Retrieved July 20, 2008, from *http://www.blackboard.com/us/index.bbb*.

Branching out: The MeSH vocabulary. (n.d.). Retrieved July 22, 2008, from the Bibliographic Services Division of the National Library of Medicine Web site: *http://www.nlm.nih.gov/bsd/disted/video/windows*.

CINAHL Information Systems. (2006, January 19). Retrieved July 22, 2008, from *http://www.cinahl.com*.

CINAHL Tutorial. (n.d.). Retrieved July 22, 2008, from the University of Florida Health Science Center Libraries Web site: *http://www.citt.ufl.edu/portfolio/cinahl*.

Dogpile. (n.d.). Retrieved July 22, 2008, from *http://www.dogpile.com*.

Dreamweaver CS3. (n.d.). Adobe Inc. Retrieved July 20, 2008, from *http://www.adobe.com/products/dreamweaver*.

ERIC. (n.d.). Retrieved July 22, 2008, from *http://www.eric.ed.gov*.

Examples of educational wikis. (n.d.). Educational Wikis. Retrieved July 22, 2008, from *http://educationalwikis.wikispaces.com/Examples+of+educational+wikis*.

Facebook. (n.d.). Retrieved July 22, 2008, from *http://www.facebook.com*.

Fair Use Checklist. (n.d.). Retrieved July 22, 2008, from the Copyright Advisory Office of Columbia University Libraries/Information Services Web site: *http://www.copyright.columbia.edu/fair-use-checklist*.

Flickr. (n.d.). Retrieved July 22, 2008, from *http://www.flickr.com/*.

FrontPage. (n.d.). Microsoft Corps. Retrieved July 17, 2008, from *http://office.microsoft.com/en-us/frontpage/default.aspx*.

Google. (n.d). Retrieved July 22, 2008, from *http://www.google.com*.

Harris, A. (n.d.). The STAIR process and searching the WWW. Retrieved July 22, 2008, from *http://www.cs.iupui.edu/~aharris/mmcc/mod2/abwww6.html*.

Hollingsworth, C. (2007, October 23). Active Learning. Retrieved July 22, 2008, from Web by Design site: *http://www.iupui.edu/~webtrain/active_learning.html.*

Hollingsworth, C. (2008, May 5). Web by Design. Retrieved July 20, 2008, from *http://www.iupui.edu/~webtrain/tutorials.html.*

How big is the Internet? (n.d.). Metamend. Retrieved July from *http://www.metamend.com/internet-growth.html.*

Librarians' Internet Index. (n.d.). Retrieved July 22, 2008, from *http://lii.org.*

LibWeb. (n.d.). Retrieved July 22, 2008, from *http://lists.webjunction.org/libweb.*

Lynch, P. J., Horton, S., & Rosenfeld, H. (2004, March 5). Alignment. Web Style Guide (2nd ed.). Retrieved July 22, 2008, from *http://webstyleguide.com/type/align.html.*

Montgomery, G. (n.d.). Color blindness: More prevalent among males. Retrieved April 16, 2008, from Howard Hughes Medical Institute Web site: *http://www.hhmi.org/senses/b130.html.*

Medline Plus. (2008, July 22). National Library of Medicine. Retrieved July 22, 2008, from *http://www.nlm.nih.gov/medlineplus.*

Moodle. (n.d.). Retrieved July 20, 2008, from *http://moodle.org.*

MySpace. (n.d.). Retrieved July 22, 2008, from *http://www.myspace.com.*

Naismith, L. (2007). Using text messaging to support administrative communication in higher education. Active Learning for Higher Education 8(2), 155–171. Retrieved July 22, 2008, from *http://alh.sagepub.com/cgi/content/abstract/8/2/155.*

Neilson, J. (1997, October 1). How users read on the Web. Retrieved July 20, 2008, from *http://www.useit.com/alertbox/9710a.html.*

NVU. (n.d.). Retrieved July 20, 2008, from *http://www.nvu.com.*

O'Reilly, T. (2005, September 30). What is Web 2.0: Design patterns and business models for the next generation of software. Retrieved July 22, 2008, from *http://www.oreillynet.com/pub/a/oreilly/tim/news/2005/09/30/what-is-web-20.html.*

SAKAI. (n.d). Retrieved July 20, 2008, from *http://sakaiproject.org.*

Second Life. (n.d.). Retrieved July 22, 2008, from *http://secondlife.com.*

Skype. (n.d.). Retrieved July 22, 2008, from *http://www.skype.com.*

Web 2.0. (n.d.). Wikipedia. Retrieved July 22, 2008, from *http://en.wikipedia.org/wiki/Web_2.0.*

WebCT. (n.d.). Retrieved July 20, 2008, from *http://www.webct.com/webct.*

Weblogg-ed. (n.d.). Retrieved July 22, 2008, from *http://weblogg-ed.com.*

WebMD. (n.d.). Retrieved July 22, 2008, from *http://www.webmd.com.*

Wikipedia. (n.d.). Retrieved July 22, 2008, from *http://www.wikipedia.org.*

Yahoo. (n.d.). Retrieved July 22, 2008, from *http://dir.yahoo.com.*

Blended learning

LEARNING OBJECTIVES

After reading this chapter, the participant will be able to:

- Identify methods for overcoming barriers in blended learning

- Discuss the role of the multigenerational classroom in blended learning

One of the newest buzzwords in staff education seems to be blended learning. Blended learning, as defined by researchers Heinze and Procter, is "learning that is facilitated by the effective combination of different modes of delivery, models of teaching and learning styles, and founded on transparent communication amongst all parties involved in a course" (2004). In recent studies, students have indicated that blended learning provides them with flexible time schedules and improved learning outcomes (Vaughan 2007). But what does blended learning mean to you, and how can it help you evolve your educational programs to be their very best?

When instituting blended learning, remember that the concepts of teaching have not changed. What has changed is the variety of resources we have at our disposal. For years, teachers have used the traditional lecture-and-test method of teaching. This method is great for auditory learners, but visual learners were left only with their class notes to use as a learning tool. The old concept holds true that learners remember 10% of what they hear, 20% of what they see, 30% of what they do, and 50% of what they hear, see, and do. So the more we can do to blend teaching methods to cover these senses, the better off we are in delivering our messages to students.

Blending learning styles

Consider the three learning preferences, which include listening (auditory learners), viewing (visual learners), and doing (kinesthetic learners), when developing a blended educational program. Figure 4.1 outlines the different teaching methods that will appeal to them; consider blending these methods to cover a wide ranging of learning preferences.

FIGURE 4.1 — Teaching methods for various learning styles

Teaching method	Type of learner
Lectures	Auditory learner
Self-learning packets	Visual learner
Online education	Visual learner
Simulation	Kinesthetic learner
Audio CDs	Auditory learner
Printouts or posters	Visual learner
Preceptor training	Kinesthetic learner

Overcoming barriers and resistance

Another question to consider before planning a blended learning program is, "What barriers are there to meeting the goal of conveying information?" Barriers can take many forms and can present significant challenges to your educational endeavors. Most often, barriers can be grouped in one of four types: physical, attitude, sensory, and cognitive. Figure 4.2 gives examples from each of these categories.

Learning how to overcome these barriers can be challenging for any educator, but understanding the concerns of your audience and conducting your research on educational methods before instituting them in the classroom can make the change smoother and help you overcome resistance from learners.

New Technology in Nursing Staff Development

FIGURE
4.2

Barriers in blended learning

Barriers	Examples
Physical	• Computer access • Quiet place to learn • Lack of learning materials (e.g., books or DVD players) • Lack of time needed to involve the learner
Attitude	• "I don't need to know this." • "I don't have time for this; I have patients to care for." • "How is this going to help me in my job?" • "What's in it for me?"
Sensory	• Hearing deficits • Visual impairments • Dexterity problems • Linguistic misinterpretations
Cognitive	• Religious or cultural conflict • Personal prejudice on the topic • Learning disabilities

Case study: Mount Auburn Hospital

A clinical nurse specialist at Mount Auburn Hospital in Cambridge, MA, was involved in implementing a pneumococcal and influenza opt-out program. This program allowed nurses to vaccinate patients based on a standing order if patients met a certain criterion. What initially seemed like a great program to improve patient care was met with a lot of resistance. Staff members asked:

- "What if the patient forgot that he or she was vaccinated before?"
- "How can I give this vaccination, and what does this standing order mean?"
- "I don't think these vaccines help. I never take them."

Armed with research on the vaccination to allay their concerns, the educator came up with a Frequently Asked Questions (FAQ) sheet that answered the staff members' questions and backed up her answers with published research findings. Blending a face-to-face inservice (for auditory learners) on the new vaccine process with a FAQ sheet with the published research findings (for visual learners) was an effective teaching strategy for staff members. Additionally, this evidence-based, blended approach helped dissolve the resistance and barriers, and the hospital achieved the goal of vaccinating patients.

In the previous case scenario, the solution worked because the educator knew her audience. It is important to know who you are trying to get your point across to when instituting new policies and practices in the blended classroom.

Blended learning also can help in overcoming another barrier you may face as an educator if your facility employs a significant number of part-time and per-diem nursing staff. As these staff members work infrequently or sporadically, it is often difficult to share information with them. Thus, the educator is required to provide education in a variety of different formats. Although a face-to-face inservice might be an effective medium that allows for question-and-answer sessions, each staff member might not always be able to attend such an inservice. In this case, it can become crucial for effective communication (and patient safety) to institute blended learning with several educational modes.

The face-to-face inservice might involve PowerPoint slides with slide handouts to ensure that the same information is provided to all; likewise, the slides can also be printed and left in the unit in a binder for staff members to review and sign off that they have read them. Some changes might be even simpler and more visual, such as posters, whereas some may be more involved, such as posting the slides on the hospital's Internet and directing staff members to them via e-mail to have them review the information.

Blended learning and the multigenerational classroom

Developing a program to meet an individual's needs can open up the possibility of learning options. There are many educational opportunities on the Internet. But what should you consider when instituting blended learning by bringing computers into the learning environment? The answer, as laid out in Figure 4.3, may depend on your students' birth dates.

FIGURE 4.3

Blended learning and the different generations

Generations	Birth dates	Technological implications
Veterans	Born between 1926 and 1945	Members of this generation did not grow up learning with computers. Their classroom environment mainly consisted of a blend of lectures, reading materials, and written tests.
Baby boomers	Born between 1946 and 1964	Often, members of this generation did not grow up with computers in their schools and may not have had them in their homes. This was still the time when typing was taught in schools on typewriters and word processors were used to type papers for school.
Generation X	Born between 1965 to 1980	This generation may have exposure to computers at home, but access to computers in the schools may have been limited.
Generation Y	Born between 1981 and 2002	This generation grew up with computers in both the home and classroom. They often spend significant time surfing the Internet and interacting with friends and family online.

When you think of blended learning, you may think of the younger generations as the ones who are adept at new technological teaching strategies. Members of Generation Y are people born between 1981 and 2002. They often grew up with computers at home and at school. They typically spend a significant amount of time surfing the Internet to get the answers they need in life, and they also use the Web socially to communicate with friends and family.

Today's Generation Yers don't even have to be home to use these resources, as they were first in line for their iPhones. For this generation, education styles without pictures and animation are often downright boring. Additionally, Yers highly value their personal time, so it's crucial to get your point across quickly, using a blended learning style that is going to make a strong, fast impression. For this reason, strategies like animated e-learning packets can work well, but they must be blended with a written test or another method that monitors the change you're trying to accomplish; that way, you're making sure that they weren't so entertained that they missed the message.

Members of the next generational group, Generation Xers, were born between 1965 and 1980. They may have had exposure to computers at home, but access to computers at school may have been limited, particularly with older Xers. Members of this generation were often known as latchkey kids who came home to an empty home as their parents were both working to make ends meet. This situation led these kids to seek entertainment in their televisions. For these reasons, try using videos with case scenarios or role-playing with your Xers.

Baby boomers were born between 1946 and 1964. This generation did not grow up with computers in school, and at home they might have had word processors or typewriters. Baby boomers were viewed as a generation of overachievers, as they often stayed in school longer than their parents.

Although self-motivated, Baby boomers now often find themselves challenged in the current world of online learning. They need a lot of reassurance that they are assimilating information and meeting objectives, so incorporating opportunities where they test their knowledge sporadically can help them gain confidence in new learning.

Members of the next generation, Veterans, were born between 1926 and 1945. Veterans are known for working hard for what they have and what they know. Their education was usually

New Technology in Nursing Staff Development

very straightforward and often involved lecture, reading, and testing. The best part of having Veterans in your audience is they are usually there because they want to be. They are motivated learners who, once you've taught them well, might serve as role models for others.

Could generation gaps create problems in the blended classroom? The reality is that many teachers are either Baby boomers or Generation Xers. There is something to be said for these generations of teachers to have and share experience with the younger generations, but perhaps these experiences should be shared through an electronic medium to reach the Generation Yers most effectively. We need to have the flexibility to meet the needs of our multigenerational work force, which might include learning preferences or barriers that differ from our own.

This approach can be used to teach basic dysrhythmia. In the following example, it's important to have a variety of resources available to help novice nurses to learn this skill.

Blended learning example: Basic dysrhythmia course

A good example of using several learning styles is in basic dysrhythmia learning options, such as at Mount Auburn Hospital in Cambridge, MA. This didactic class reviews the defining characteristics of each rhythm with practice strips after each section: sinus, atrial, junctional, and blocks, as well as a mix-up of practice strips to help integrate the information obtained in each section. This is a great modality to start with because it involves a live teacher to answer questions such as, "Why isn't it this rhythm?"

If learners leave this course still unsure of how to define characteristics of the rhythms, an online continuing education program has proven useful. This program reviews the same information that's in the live course but may help more visual learners or learners who just need more practice to gain confidence.

At this point, it's usually time to start applying what has been learned into practice. You can do so by using competency-based checklists, which are skill-specific lists of knowledge or skills that novice nurses must be able to perform to be deemed competent by their preceptors. For the novice, the checklists set clear expectations for what they need to know, and they provide standardization for our preceptors in determining competence.

Once staff members have an understanding of basic rhythms, some units at Mount Auburn will use a "Strip of the Week" technique, in which more challenging rhythms are posted. Staff members are given a few days to come to their own conclusions regarding the rhythms, and the answer is later posted along with a description of why it met the defining characteristics of the rhythm.

The last option for more experienced students is EKG Wave Maven, which is an Internet-based program that requires the student to integrate EKG interpretation into case scenarios and asks students for their best response. As you can see from Figure 4.4, you can use an interpretation checklist to determine staff competency in a given subject—in this case, basic dysrhythmia. With some topics, you sometimes need different levels of teaching materials as the student grows from novice to expert.

For independent learners, it may be most effective to compose a tool that includes a reference list of materials you used to put the class together. Note which materials would be particularly beneficial if they need additional practice or which material presents the information differently.

New Technology in Nursing Staff Development

FIGURE
4.4

Basic dysrhythmia interpretation

How competency was met:			
O	Observation	P	Patient feedback
CH	Chart audit	S	Simulation
Q	Question/answer	PR	Peer review
CS	Case study	T	Test

Performance criteria	Validated		
	Yes	No	By:
1. Successfully completes basic dysrhythmia exam score			
2. Demonstrates appropriate lead placement for monitoring			
3. Demonstrates understanding of central station operation			
4. Demonstrates understanding of PR interval, QRS complex, and T waves			
5. Demonstrates accuracy of interval measurement PR interval, QRS complex, and QT interval			
6. States appropriate documentation time frames			
7. Demonstrates ability to accurately identify rhythms			
8. Demonstrates knowledge of appropriate therapeutic interventions to treat dysrhythmias			

Comments: _____

Validated by: _____

Date: _____

Source: Mount Auburn Hospital, Cambridge, MA. Used with permission.

Choosing methods to blend

By now you may be wondering, "Which teaching styles should be blended with which?" There is a reason why the blending of lecture and testing has stood the test of time: It is based on fundamentals of communication. For effective communication to occur, the message must:

- Be conveyed

- Be received by the learner

- Ignite a response

- Be understood

As seen in Figure 4.5, each phase of communication can be accomplished or monitored by instituting the following teaching/learning strategies.

Because learning involves changing a student's knowledge, skills, or attitudes regarding a topic, it is important not only to share information with your students through blended learning but also to check whether you've met your learning objectives of change. Information can be conveyed via lecture, reading, computer, demonstration, role playing, or case studies; the important thing is to then use another teaching style alongside the original method to validate understanding. To do so, integrate test questions into a game such as *Jeopardy*; this approach can add fun into learning and help you engage your students.

New Technology in Nursing Staff Development

FIGURE
4.5

The message must be conveyed	Methods for conveying information can include: • Lectures • Reading materials • Online information • Posters
The message must be received	Getting a message received by learners is often more difficult than conveying it. In nursing, we make strategic decisions on whether the message can be conveyed while the nurse is on the unit or not. On-unit education usually needs to be short or distractions make it impossible for the message to be received. This is where online and blended learning can help learners effectively receive information without the distractions of physical surroundings.
The message must ignite a response	Education is often used with the goal of changing something; therefore, it's important to understand the desired change and to measure it to determine whether there was a response to your educational endeavors.
The message must be understood	Educators often forget this critical step; a blended learning approach can be especially effective at this step as you attempt to answer the question, "How do I know they got the message?" This can be done through: • Simulated procedures • Case scenarios • Games

Case studies also can be helpful when you're trying to integrate new actions into practice. In the case study, you can give your students a situation in which you want to new behavior to be incorporated.

When the goal is to teach a new skill, the best validation technique is to have the learner simulate the skill. Lastly, if you're trying to affect a new attitude about a patient population, role-playing can be a fun way for staff members to depict very challenging situations. Because role-playing involves thinking on your feet, the teaching really needs to be adopted to show up quickly in a role-play. The best aspect of this method is that even if the role-play does not validate understanding, it is another teaching moment in the classroom.

Evaluating your options

Now that we've discussed the ins and outs of blended learning, let's take a look at how you can evaluate this teaching option and determine whether it's right for your organization.

Deciding on the right technology

As you determine whether to institute blended learning in your classroom, be sure to ask yourself the following questions:

- **Is your organization ready electronically?** Are there computers available to staff members for education? Do your computers have CD capability? Do you have DVD players on the floors?

- **Are your educators proficient in electronic media?** Some of your educators who are not accustomed to veering from the traditional classroom setting may not be proficient in blended learning, even while they are teaching tech savvy students who love it. You may need to do some up front work by explaining this generational gap to your leadership to get some upfront finances to send you to computer classes you'll need to be successful.

- **Are your staff members proficient in using computers?** Are they using computers to do their everyday work? If you think there could be a computer phobia in your organization, do you have the information technology resources within the organization to help staff members?

Justifying your resources

As a change agent in your organization, it is important to strategize how to move your organization forward so that the entire organization can grow. When justifying the time and resources needed to institute blended learning, consider the following strategies:

- **Get yourself and your education team ready.** Enroll in some computer education. Use your organization's information technology experts and/or media experts. These efforts will be key when justifying that blended learning should be instituted.

- **Give examples of ways projects could be adapted into blended learning.** For example, discuss how blended learning can assist in the orientation of agency or travel staff members. To help orient supplemental staff members to your organization in a time-efficient manner, put together a CD program with the cognitive information about what is specific to your organization with a quiz to validate the integration of knowledge. Projects such as these can play a big part in justifying blended learning.

Obtaining administrative buy-in

When advocating to your administration for the electronic media access you need for blended learning, you must listen to what is important for you organization to improve upon and finding e-learning media that will support it.

Once you start demonstrating what staff members can learn this way, you can generate the evidence you need to support the financial expenditure it might take. Show that it could be time-efficient for the hospital educators by showing your administrators a cost-benefit analysis.

Obtaining staff buy-in

When attempting to get staff members on board for blended learning, one method is to start small and let blended learning grow within your organization. For example, you may want to integrate this approach into your continuing education programs. Staff members who attend continuing education are often especially interested in the topic you are teaching. They may welcome the variety of learning styles presented in a blended learning approach program.

Additionally, using the face-to-face classroom initially for blended learning may be the way to get staff buy-in; you'll have the opportunity to support them with any technical aspects concerning accessing information. Then, when you ask your nurses to access online information for education, they feel confident and comfortable.

Conclusion

The challenge in healthcare is that we are usually trying to create change over time. For this reason, it's sometimes important to develop monitors that units can use to measure the change until it has become the culture. Blended learning will help to involve and engage your learners; it will make your education more entertaining and exciting. Thus, it will result in charge that stays. Not only that, but it will also help you, the educator, successfully get your message across to your multigenerational students and reassure you that your message has been received.

References

Heinze, A., and C. Procter. 2004. "Reflections on the use of blended learning." Salford, United Kingdom: University of Salford.

Vaughan, N. 2007. "Perspectives on blended learning in higher education." *International Journal on E-Learning* 6(1): 81–94.

Simulation

After reading this chapter, the
participant will be able to:

- List the benefits of using
  simulation as a staff
  training tool

Simulation as a teaching strategy for healthcare disciplines has grown exponentially since the beginning of
the 21st century. The complexity of healthcare has
forced healthcare institutions, academic and service
alike, to consider new ways of training and developing
nurses and other healthcare practitioners. Simulation
has enjoyed a recent surge of interest and development
as evidenced by major capital investments in simulation
tools, equipment, and centers. New graduates are
coming to work with simulation experience from their
academic programs. Here, we'll explore the background
and some how-to aspects of simulation as a teaching
strategy so you can discover this training method as an
option for your institution.

What is simulation?

Educational simulation offers the opportunity for
learners to "fulfill assigned roles ... in an environment
that models reality" (Hertel and Millis 2002). Within
nursing education, simulation has been a pedagogical
strategy for decades. Role-playing and skills lab
activities (Gomez and Gomez 1987), often using task
trainers and static mannequins, are older simulation
strategies within nursing education that are still

commonly in use. Traditional skills labs across the country are integrating simulation to create clinical learning centers.

Microsimulation has historically been used by the military to simulate battlefield situations and the aviation industry for training purposes; it has since been adapted for use in healthcare settings. However, nursing education programs, both in service and academic settings, have refocused on simulation as pedagogy, especially with the recent advent of computerized mannequins, also known as high-fidelity patient simulators. Simulation, however, is more than just a mannequin (Seropian, Brown, Gavilanes, and Driggers 2004).

Characteristics of simulation strategies

Educators often use terms such as technology and fidelity to describe the characteristics of simulation used as pedagogy. Technology generally refers to the level of computerization that the simulation strategy requires. For example, the computerized mannequins that breathe, have pulses with realistic anatomy and physiology, and can verbalize with appropriate microphone setup are considered high-tech, whereas a role-play of a case conference requires no more technology than a typical conference room has. The latter would be described as low-tech. An example of a mid-tech simulation tool is a mannequin that has breath and heart sounds but lacks excursion of the chest.

The degree of fidelity—that is, the degree of realism that engages the learner—is much more important than the level of technology. The primary reason for using simulation as pedagogy is to provide learners with practice in a realistic environment as possible in order to gain confidence, thereby increasing the potential for safer patient care experiences (Salas, Wilson, Burke, and Priest 2005). Simulations may be considered low fidelity, as in the case of task trainers (e.g., a left- or right-sided rubberized gluteus maximus with a reddened area, indicating skin breakdown, used for wound care training) or virtual reality trainers, such as a laparoscopic surgery trainer; or high fidelity, as in the case of computerized mannequins (e.g., a simulated patient in which the patient has breath sounds, cardiac sounds and pulses, converses with the nurse about his increasing shortness of breath, and whose chest rises and falls with each breath).

Beyond the type of simulation tool, the level of fidelity can be enhanced by attending to the details within the learning environment. A high-fidelity simulation session includes the equipment and environmental cues that engage the learner in practicing communication, aspects of team-work, and/or the intended learning objectives. This is sometimes referred to as psychological fidelity. Even in the absence of a high-tech human patient simulator or other forms of simulation, fidelity can be improved by implementing a policy that requires learners to wear practice attire (e.g., scrubs, white lab jackets) and any personal protective equipment required by the situation. The policy also should ensure that the practice setting closely resembles the actual scenario's environment, such as a patient care room. In addition to enhancing the fidelity, such a policy helps participants bring a level of professionalism and maturity to their roles.

Why use simulation?

The current status of the healthcare world leaves much room for simulation as an effective teaching tool. The benefits to simulation technology are numerous; let's explore a few of the ways that simulation in education can improve the nursing profession.

Expanded role of the nurse in a shortage

Healthcare is more complex than ever before. Patients are sicker and stay in hospitals for shorter times because of rising healthcare costs. The demand for nurses who think clearly and appropriately in clinical situations is greater than ever before (Tanner 2005). In addition, there is currently a nursing shortage, predicted to be more severe and longer lasting than previous shortages (Johnson and Johnson 2003).

In the academic realm, nursing education programs are increasingly challenged to graduate more nurses in shorter time frames in order to address the deficit while constantly competing with other programs for clinical practice settings that give students the experiences they need. Educational and service settings are collaborating to produce in nurses the excellent clinical thinking that the marketplace requires (Porter-O'Grady 2001). However, some observers note that today's graduates are not ready to practice fully upon completion of their educational program (del Bueno 2005). Other healthcare professions, such as medicine, are also experiencing challenges for clinical practice opportunities, such as the implementation of the 80-hour work week for residents (Accreditation Council for Graduate Medical Education, 2008). Simulation offers an opportunity to address these limitations, especially as interprofessional team training grows.

In response, institutions have implemented comprehensive orientation and mentoring programs (American Nurses Credentialing Center 2008), and institutional accrediting bodies require individual development plans for new hires and ongoing staff development for more experienced nurses (The Joint Commission 2008). Many new nurse graduates who have had simulation integrated into their nursing education expect to train with simulation in their professional positions.

The Institute of Medicine's (IOM) now infamous report, identifying that nearly 100,000 patients per year die of healthcare provider errors in the United States, has served as a crucial mandate to improve education for healthcare professionals (IOM 1999). In order to achieve better outcomes and meet regulatory requirements, healthcare institutions have elevated patient safety to the highest priority. The focus on teamwork has been identified as one of the keys to patient safety (IOM 2003). Simulation can be an effective means for integrating new graduate nurses into practice settings, reinforcing ongoing education, and helping them to work in interprofessional teams.

What simulation offers learners

Colleagues and/or executives may question the value of simulation, especially when it appears to affect productivity or challenges staffing. Although mannequin-based simulation is relatively new, simulation provides an opportunity for learners to construct, enhance, and reinforce their knowledge in a healthcare context through hands-on experience. Early educators, such as Piaget (1969) and Dewey (1933), recognized the strengths of contextual learning, which implies learning about culture as well as practice. This type of learning is best done in a realistic situation with peers and facilitators, such as staff developers or preceptors, thus forming a kind of learning community. Kolb (1984) touted experiential learning as a means for fully grasping new concepts. As a means for bridging the theory/practice gap, Schön (1987) further described the development of professional artistry through coaching by more mature practitioners. Simulation has the potential to integrate all of these important educational concepts (Lasater 2007a).

Formative vs. summative assessment

One of the advantages of simulation is that it provides an opportunity to integrate the cognitive, psychomotor, and affective learning necessary for professional preparation (Lasater 2007a) and ongoing education in a safe practice setting. For this reason, it is recommended that simulation should be used for formative assessment rather than for summative assessment. The latter is usually associated with high-stakes consequences, including potential failure and loss of confidence. If the outcome of simulation provides a grade or some other form of summative evaluation, this evaluation becomes the focus for the participant and distracts from his or her comfort with practicing and learning. It is crucial, therefore, to create a safe environment if learning is the goal of simulation.

Simulation choices for different outcomes

The desired learning outcome for staff development education should guide the choice of simulation strategy. For example, if the primary outcome for training is for the nurse to develop competency in starting IVs, the most straightforward and least expensive form of simulation is a task trainer, such as an IV arm. If, however, the desired learning outcome is to help nurses learn to work in crisis situations as part of the emergency department team, a simulation scenario using a computerized mannequin and members from the entire team may be the most appropriate form of simulation. When nurses need to learn to be more active members in a case conference or to deal with a combative patient, role-play may be the most desirable form. Therefore, it is essential to have intentional learning outcomes for the simulation and to discuss the options during planning.

The planning of simulation sessions should be done by content experts as well as nurse preceptors and other staff members who have responsibility for the learners. If there are specific courses that new hires attend, the idea of spiraling the learning or increasing the complexity with ongoing development should be considered (Harden and Stamper 1999).

Different forms of simulation

Once the desired learning outcome has been determined, the educator should carefully consider the available simulation options. This section details the primary forms of simulation that are in current use: task trainers, microsimulation, role-play, and mannequin-based simulation. The advantages and disadvantages of each form are considered as well. Because high-fidelity mannequins are relatively new and have much to offer for education and practice, this chapter will focus on this form of simulation.

Task trainers

If the expected outcome for learning is psychomotor skill attainment or increased expertise, the appropriate choice of simulation tool is a task trainer (Jeffries and Rogers 2007). Task trainers are different body parts used for focused training and skill practice. Examples include tracheostomy and airway heads, IV arms, wound care models, Foley catheter insertion models, injection models, and central venous catheter models.

The clear advantage of task trainers is that they offer an uncomplicated focus for learning and practice, without all of the distractions and details that accompany entrance into a patient room. They are available at a relatively low cost. In addition, they can be transported and used almost anywhere, with little human support. The disadvantage is that they focus on an isolated task without the realism, patient communication, or other environmental aspects that add up to the complete patient care experience.

Microsimulation

Microsimulation is a type of program that can be installed on a computer for learners to practice working through cases. After spending "real time" with a given scenario, learners get feedback from an online debriefing guide focused on areas that were not done completely or accurately (Christensen 2006).

One of the biggest advantages of microsimulation is that it is a self-guided opportunity that allows learners to spend the time needed to work through practice cases; it may also provide evaluation information (Billings and Halstead 1998). Although there is not an instructor or manager looking over learners' shoulders or giving them time pressure, the cases still run in a real-time format. Some of the programs offer management systems that allow the educator to note the learners' scores and/or create a report of completion or a list of those who may need to do more study.

One disadvantage for some will be the time needed to learn how to use the program before they are able to move on to make clinical judgments in the real-time scenario. Another disadvantage is the isolated nature of the microsimulation; there is no opportunity to learn from other learners and/or a facilitator. Another consideration is that the sessions are usually scored. This may work well for a learner who wants to keep trying until they reach perfection but does not ensure concept retention. Finally, unless the material is mandated as part of a training session, it is unlikely that learners will choose to do it in their free time.

Role-play

Role-play involves setting up a situation in which participants play specific characters. These situations range from a two-person role-play (e.g., where a nurse is teaching a patient about diabetic foot care) to a multiple-person role-play, such as a multidisciplinary case conference with the patient, family members, and a variety of healthcare practitioners. A role-play may involve a fairly constructed script or be implemented on the fly with some pivotal scripted moments that direct how it unfolds.

Standardized patients. Standardized patients are actors who are hired to play the roles of patients and are given personality descriptions of their characters, along with scripts of responses to scenario actions. Historically, standardized patients have been used to practice taking health histories or doing physical assessments (Jenkins et al 2006; Rentschler et al 2007). The interviews and examinations take place in rooms that are similar to clinic examining rooms, which provides environmental fidelity. The pay for actors varies based on the nature of the examination, with higher pay for more invasive exams, such as gynecological. Clearly, policies need to be in place to safeguard both examiners and patients; many centers develop elaborate ways to videotape the interactions, with the possibility of real-time viewing by faculty. Some allow a coach or peers to be in the examination room for support and for peer learning. Usually, standardized patients are trained to offer feedback to learners after the role-play.

The fidelity of the setting is a real advantage to this form of role-play, and most healthcare institutions can easily accommodate it. However, if special remodeling is required to create a center with a high level of audio/visual support, the project can prove to be a major expense, with the additional costs of the actors.

Standardized participants. Some institutions are using more casual actors, such as peers or staff developers, as standardized participants who are given character descriptions. Because the actors are often familiar to those engaged in the case, environmental and psychological fidelity must enhance this type of role play for it to be most effective. The chief advantage of using standardized participants is that they are generally part of the learning environment already, so they do not require additional payment.

Advantages and disadvantages of role-play

Role-play, in whatever form, offers some important advantages. It rarely involves any technology, so it is a simple, low-cost alternative and provides some options for patient cases that mannequin-based simulation does not. For example, mannequins do not offer a high degree of fidelity when communication is the primary focus, such as in an interview with a patient who has schizoaffective disorder, or where a group is involved, such as delivering bad news to a patient and family. The primary disadvantage of role-play is that some participants may have difficulty suspending disbelief to embrace their roles, thereby decreasing the situation's fidelity. Well-planned role-plays with a clear purpose will facilitate the psychological fidelity for most. Staffing challenges and other time demands also may make it difficult to gather a group to implement role-play cases effectively. Gaining the cooperation and buy-in of department leaders is critical for overcoming this barrier.

Mannequin-based simulation

As previously mentioned, there are low-, mid-, and high-fidelity training and learning opportunities in simulation, even within the types of mannequins:

- **Low-fidelity mannequins,** sometimes referred to as static or passive, have long been used when teaching and practicing cardiopulmonary resuscitation. Resusci-Annie and other similar mannequins are familiar to most nurses from CPR training. Often, these mannequins are upper bodies only.

- **Mid-fidelity mannequins,** also referred to as basic simulators, have full bodies and limited characteristics, such as heart and lung sounds or birthing capabilities (Spunt 2007).

- **High-fidelity mannequins** have programmable capability to respond to interventions with actions, such as changing vital signs or lung sounds, and have gained recent popularity due to their physiological realism and flexibility for use in a wide variety of settings.

The advantages of mannequin-based simulation are endless in terms of the possibilities for training and practice. Depending on the location of the simulation center, the ability to bring the patient to the nursing staff not only helps the realism but also brings the potential to get more staff members involved. In addition to the staffing and scheduling challenges discussed earlier, one of the biggest disadvantages of mannequin-based simulation is access to dedicated space in the practice setting.

   New Technology in Nursing Staff Development

The logistical considerations and challenges with set up and storage can be substantial. If there is no dedicated simulation space and the facility is relying on in situ (hospital room) simulation, it is crucial to check out the location ahead of time to ensure that the outlets are in the correct locations and determine how best to set up the session. Simulations can occur in a variety of settings, including the simulation center, in situ, classroom, or at the bedside. Each has its own strengths and barriers for implementation; again, consider the goals of the learners and the overall objectives, along with physical capacity. Whatever the setting, it is critical to use checklists to ensure smooth operation and flow of the session; an example of such a checklist can be found in Figure 5.1.

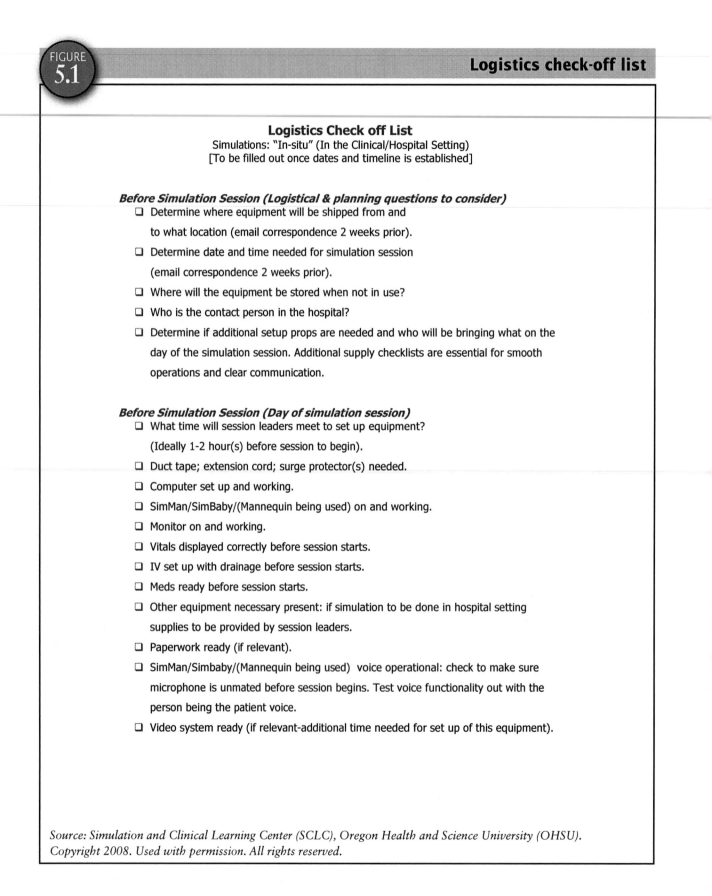

FIGURE
5.1

Logistics check-off list

Logistics Check off List
Simulations: "In-situ" (In the Clinical/Hospital Setting)
[To be filled out once dates and timeline is established]

Before Simulation Session (Logistical & planning questions to consider)
- ❏ Determine where equipment will be shipped from and
  to what location (email correspondence 2 weeks prior).
- ❏ Determine date and time needed for simulation session
  (email correspondence 2 weeks prior).
- ❏ Where will the equipment be stored when not in use?
- ❏ Who is the contact person in the hospital?
- ❏ Determine if additional setup props are needed and who will be bringing what on the
  day of the simulation session. Additional supply checklists are essential for smooth
  operations and clear communication.

Before Simulation Session (Day of simulation session)
- ❏ What time will session leaders meet to set up equipment?
  (Ideally 1-2 hour(s) before session to begin).
- ❏ Duct tape; extension cord; surge protector(s) needed.
- ❏ Computer set up and working.
- ❏ SimMan/SimBaby/(Mannequin being used) on and working.
- ❏ Monitor on and working.
- ❏ Vitals displayed correctly before session starts.
- ❏ IV set up with drainage before session starts.
- ❏ Meds ready before session starts.
- ❏ Other equipment necessary present: if simulation to be done in hospital setting
  supplies to be provided by session leaders.
- ❏ Paperwork ready (if relevant).
- ❏ SimMan/Simbaby/(Mannequin being used) voice operational: check to make sure
  microphone is unmated before session begins. Test voice functionality out with the
  person being the patient voice.
- ❏ Video system ready (if relevant-additional time needed for set up of this equipment).

*Source: Simulation and Clinical Learning Center (SCLC), Oregon Health and Science University (OHSU).
Copyright 2008. Used with permission. All rights reserved.*

Many institutions, both academic and service, are establishing centers that may have one or more simulation complex, sometimes referred to as simulation apartments, each of which includes the simulation theater itself, a control room behind a one-way mirror, and a debriefing room. However, that is not the only option, and therefore, it is important to think outside of the box. Lack of space or designated simulation apartment should not deter from integrating simulation as a learning tool.

Within nursing staff education, in situ simulation—taking the human patient simulator into the patient care setting—is often the most ideal (Rall, Stricker, Reddersen, Zieger, and Dieckmann 2008). This option is great from an environmental perspective because nurses already know how to (or need to practice) acquiring all of the equipment needed during a patient care encounter. This situation allows the nurses to focus more on communication, teamwork, and clinical judgment, along with the potential resource management challenges that may arise. Additionally, in situ simulation offers the unique opportunity to test institutional systems, policies, and procedures.

Other location options include the classroom or lecture room setting (Seropian, Dillman, Lasater, and Gavilanes 2007), running the mannequin from a laptop as a patient care replication on the stage. This option is most effective for teaching large groups about the dramatic effects of certain drugs on vital signs, for example. Others have used the in situ setup near a bedside with the mannequin to run several small groups of students through an unfolding case. For example, two nurses at a time care for the patient while the staff development specialist runs the computer on a bedside stand nearby; the action stops for discussion and reorientation and then resumes, with another dyad taking over the patient care and so forth.

Clearly, psychological fidelity is compromised in this situation, but it may be used effectively for those new to mannequin-based simulation or to beginning students because it can diffuse the mystique of the mannequin and demonstrate how it works. It can also provide an important opportunity to practice handoffs, such as giving end-of-shift reports. Taking simulation "on the road" outside of a permanent location requires that the room and technology setup be checked in advance and that the facilitator has all of the needed equipment to implement in situ simulation. A checklist can facilitate these important considerations.

Acquiring simulation scenarios. Nursing scenarios suitable for use in simulation are available for purchase, often from the mannequin manufacturers. Limited preprogrammed scenarios may come with the mannequins. However, writing your own scenarios—tailored to the institution, types of patients, or greatest quality improvement issues—may offer a higher-quality product. In other words, before investing large sums of money in someone else's scenarios, be very clear about the purposes and expectations surrounding the use of mannequin-based simulations. If the primary purpose is to enhance clinical thinking in complex situations, a conceptual framework for development, debriefing, and evaluation of the simulations may be very useful in order to create scenarios that support clinical thinking. One such framework is the adapted Model of Clinical Judgment (Tanner 2006), which is evidence-based and describes the contextual thinking behind nurses' clinical judgments. This model, which Tanner has adapted from the original, is seen below in Figure 5.2.

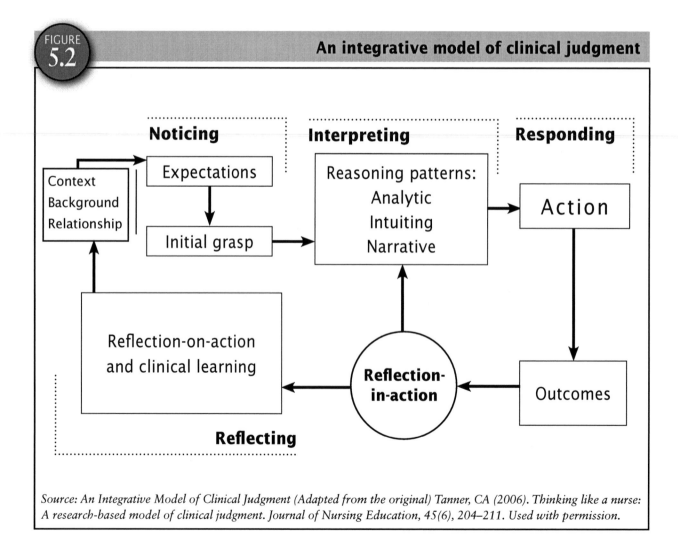

FIGURE 5.2

An integrative model of clinical judgment

Source: An Integrative Model of Clinical Judgment (Adapted from the original) Tanner, CA (2006). Thinking like a nurse: A research-based model of clinical judgment. Journal of Nursing Education, 45(6), 204–211. Used with permission.

A closer look at the model offers a snapshot of the complexity of nurses' thinking. The context of care, the life and professional experiences the nurse brings to the care setting, and his or her relationship with the patient set up expectations of what the nurse may notice upon his or her initial contact. Based on those expectations, the nurse, depending on his or her background, may quickly grasp if a patient situation demands attention or intervention. In other words, the Noticing phase of the model is critical to what follows.

Interpreting involves a complex array of reasoning patterns, including but not limited to analytic, intuitive, and narrative, and often almost simultaneously (Tanner 2006). These patterns allow the nurse to come to some conclusions about Responding or taking action, which produces patient outcomes and sets the stage for Reflecting, both in-action (as the patient outcomes unfold) and on-action (after the action is complete). Most clinical learning occurs in this final phase of clinical judgment; this notion of reflection being the key to learning is well supported by the learning theorists mentioned earlier and others (Boud, Keogh, and Walker 1985; Dewey 1933; Schön 1987) as well as by nursing theorists and educators (Benner 1984; Benner, Tanner, and Chesla 1996; Cato, Lasater, and Peeples in press; Craft 2005; Lasater and Nielsen, in press; Murphy 2004; Nielsen, Stragnell, and Jester 2007).

Developed through another evidence-based process, dimensions of clinical judgment—which describe what is meant by effective Noticing, Interpreting, Responding, and Reflecting—provide useful foci for implementing the Model of Clinical Judgment in developing or tailoring scenarios. They help ensure that the scenarios meet the intended learning outcomes and inform the debriefing and evaluation processes (outlined later in Figure 5.4). These processes will be described in the next section.

Strategies for implementation

Implementation of scenarios requires an organized approach. According to some experts, the full-scale high-fidelity simulation experience offers three learning opportunities: one for the participants in the scenario, one for the observers of the scenario, and another for all of the above as they engage in the debriefing of the scenario (Seropian, Brown, Gavilanes, and Driggers 2004). The intended learning outcomes should always guide (a) the development or adaptation of the scenario; (b) the designated preparation for the participants, if any; (c) the actual implementation of the scenario, including the computer set up, scripting and costuming for the actors, the additional components of the scenario, such as medications, equipment, and moulage (defined as a form of make-up, often used in a theatrical setting, which can also be used in a clinical setting or with standardized patients); and (d) how the scenario will be debriefed.

Ensuring the scenario runs well is most easily accomplished using a template and checklists. A template provides the overview of the entire scenario, including the intended learning outcomes, the details of the characters and their communication, and the setup and special equipment needs. Such a tool serves as a script and allows the facilitator to organize the scenario. Samples of such templates are available in most books about simulation; one is shown in Figure 5.3.

FIGURE
5.3 **Sample scenario template**

Generic blank template

Scenario name:

Designed for:

I. Objectives (possible suggestions):

I I. Patient data

Patient name:

Age:

Case history:

Summary:

Details:

Physical exam:

Kg   HR   BP   RR   O2Sat

   Chest:
   CV:
   Abdomen:
   Head:
   MSK:
   T:

FIGURE 5.3 — **Sample scenario template (cont.)**

III. Case flow and possible outcomes:

Event	Possible actions	Outcome
		THEN:
		THEN:
		THEN:
		THEN:
		THEN:
		THEN:
		THEN:
		THEN:

IV. Equipment/setting:

V. Actors:

VI. Program:

VII. Debriefing:

VIII. References:

Source: SimHealth Consultants. 2008. Used with permission. All rights reserved.

New Technology in Nursing Staff Development

Perhaps the most critical component of determining how the scenario unfolds involves the cues that the simulation facilitator will use to ensure that the intended learning outcomes are met. These cues may involve the patient's communication, some physiological changes or lab results that are written into the scenario, or the appearance of an actor playing the physician or a family member who, in context, helps to direct the action. Considering what materials will be available to the learners ahead of time, whether for preparation or charts (including doctor's orders), adds to the fidelity of the situation and helps frame the context for the learners.

Preparation for the learners. The facilitator must decide how the learners will be prepared for the simulation activities. If there will be multiple scenarios in a session, learners may be given a list of patients and their diagnoses with which to mentally prepare. Perhaps learners will know only that they will be working in a scenario during which a crisis occurs or where teamwork is critical. Determining how participants will be in the scenario, how many will be observing the scenario, and who will be involved in debriefing is another key decision.

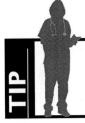

TIP

Unless the scenario is focused on an interprofessional team event, such as a resuscitation, we recommend the ideal number of active participants be two or three with a clearly designated leader.

Learners need an orientation and time to look over the environment in order to identify where equipment and medications are and how things work. Simulation facilitators should show them the features of the mannequin; for example, the mannequins have certain areas that are safe for infusion or injection. Some of the older versions may have certain points on the chest where apical pulses or lung sounds are best heard. Learners may want to time to explore and handle equipment, such as monitors or infusion pumps that are part of the environment. The use of the telephone—who can be contacted, how to get help—is an important part of the orientation.

Implementation of the scenario. Checklists for the scenario implementation are useful so that no detail is forgotten, thereby adding to the realism. The equipment (e.g., Foley catheters and bags, IVs, and medications) required to accurately portray the scenario must be prepared and set up in advance. The appearance of the mannequin may vary by gender (e.g., wigs, clothing, makeup, false eyelashes, hats), by age (e.g., clothing, stuffed animals, high-tech gadgets), or by condition (e.g., rashes, pregnancy, blood clots, created through moulage, which can add elements of detail or medical injuries and bruises that are relevant to a simulation case) (Alinier 2008). The manufacturers are usually the best resource to learn the computer programming and functionality of the mannequins; most mannequin vendors will offer training and ongoing support, which may add cost to the price.

Debriefing. Debriefing has been defined as "a process in which people who have had an experience are led through a purposive discussion of that experience" (Lederman 1992). Many students and facilitators of simulation have identified that debriefing is where the real learning is cemented (Hertel and Millis 2002; Lasater 2007a). Seropian et al. (2004) state debriefing as a peer group or learning community is the third learning opportunity of a simulation scenario. By contrast, debriefing also carries the most risk for the learner if not properly facilitated. Facilitating the discussion of learners' experiences in debriefing takes practice and should focus on active discovery on the part of the learners. It is often useful to have a secondary debriefer to facilitate from the side in order to have another set of ears and eyes during this crucial activity.

There are many resources for learning about debriefing, but one relatively simple overview centers on three aspects of learners' experience:

- The emotions elicited from them as human beings

- The activities and facts embedded in their roles during the scenario

- The learning for them as professional nurses (Hertel and Millis 2002)

The more realistic the simulation is, the greater the emotional impact. It is almost impossible to grasp the learning from the situation when learners are engulfed in emotion. In order to move forward, the emotion needs to be acknowledged. Discussing the perceptions of what happened with the learners allows them to recall the order of the events and gives opportunities to identify the critical decision points in their thinking. Last but not least, it helps all of the learners, participants and observers, make the connections and learn from what went well and what did not. Evidence-based dimensions of clinical judgment are outlined in Figure 5.4. If the intended learning outcomes are focused on clinical judgment, for example, the dimensions of clinical judgment (Lasater 2007b) can serve as a guide for formulating questions to facilitate the debriefing (see Figure 5.5):

FIGURE
5.4

Evidence-based dimensions of clinical judgment

Phase of clinical judgment	Clinical judgment dimension
Noticing	Focused observation Recognizing deviations from expected patterns Information seeking
Interpreting	Prioritizing data Making sense of data
Responding	Calm, confident manner Clear communication Well-planned intervention/flexibility Being skillful
Reflecting	Reflection/self-analysis Commitment to improvement

Source: Kathie Lasater. Used with permission (Lasater, 2007b).

FIGURE 5.5 **Sample debriefing questions by dimension to foster clinical judgment**

Phase of clinical judgment	Clinical judgment dimension	Sample debriefing questions
Noticing	• Focused observation	What did you first notice about the client?
	• Recognizing deviations from expected patterns	How was what you noticed different than what you expected?
	• Information seeking	What other information would you like to know?
Interpreting	• Prioritizing data	What was the most important priority for this client?
	• Making sense of data	With what evidence did you determine the priority?
Responding	• Calm, confident manner	How do you think you gained the client's trust?
	• Clear communication	What did you convey to the client about what you were doing?
	• Well-planned intervention/flexibility	What factors affected your choice of intervention?
	• Being skillful	How did your response compare to the standard of care?
Reflecting	• Reflection/self-analysis	What went well? Why?
	• Commitment to improvement	What would you do differently if you had it to do over?

Source: Kathie Lasater. Used with permission (Lasater, 2007b).

Evaluation. If learning is the focus of simulation in your institution, beware of correcting learners during a scenario, making evaluation a rigid outcome, or using language that implies there is one right way. The facilitator should gently guide the learners' evaluation of the experience. Even a simple question at the end of the debriefing such as "What are you taking away from today's session?" or "What did you learn today that you can use in your practice?" can help them reflect on their experience and safely identify an important concept, as well as set the stage for further evaluation and reflection.

If clinical thinking is the goal of the session, the facilitator must help the learner recognize that such thinking is complex and a developmental process. Seeing oneself on a trajectory of development can help learners to self-evaluate as well as set goals. A developmental rubric can be an effective tool for reflecting on evidence-based clinical judgment and setting goals, which are outlined in the clinical judgment rubric found in Figure 5.6.

FIGURE
5.6

Lasater clinical judgment rubric

Noticing and Interpreting

Effective NOTICING involves:	Exemplary	Accomplished	Developing	Beginning
Focused Observation	Focuses observation appropriately; regularly observes and monitors a wide variety of objective and subjective data to uncover any useful information	Regularly observes/monitors a variety of data, including both subjective and objective; most useful information is noticed, may miss the most subtle signs	Attempts to monitor a variety of subjective and objective data, but is overwhelmed by the array of data; focuses on the most obvious data, missing some important information	Confused by the clinical situation and the amount/type of data; observation is not organized and important data is missed, and/or assessment errors are made
Recognizing Deviations from Expected Patterns	Recognizes subtle patterns and deviations from expected patterns in data and uses these to guide the assessment	Recognizes most obvious patterns and deviations in data and uses these to continually assess	Identifies obvious patterns and deviations, missing some important information; unsure how to continue the assessment	Focuses on one thing at a time and misses most patterns/deviations from expectations; misses opportunities to refine the assessment
Information Seeking	Assertively seeks information to plan intervention: carefully collects useful subjective data from observing the client and from interacting with the client and family	Actively seeks subjective information about the client's situation from the client and family to support planning interventions; occasionally does not pursue important leads	Makes limited efforts to seek additional information from the client/family; often seems not to know what information to seek and/or pursues unrelated information	Is ineffective in seeking information; relies mostly on objective data; has difficulty interacting with the client and family and fails to collect important subjective data
Effective INTERPRETING involves:	Exemplary	Accomplished	Developing	Beginning
Prioritizing Data	Focuses on the most relevant and important data useful for explaining the client's condition	Generally focuses on the most important data and seeks further relevant information, but also may try to attend to less pertinent data	Makes an effort to prioritize data and focus on the most important, but also attends to less relevant/useful data	Has difficulty focusing and appears not to know which data are most important to the diagnosis; attempts to attend to all available data
Making Sense of Data	Even when facing complex, conflicting or confusing data, is able to (1) note and make sense of patterns in the client's data, (2) compare these with known patterns (from the nursing knowledge base, research, personal experience, and intuition), and (3) develop plans for interventions that can be justified in terms of their likelihood of success	In most situations, interprets the client's data patterns and compares with known patterns to develop an intervention plan and accompanying rationale; the exceptions are rare or complicated cases where it is appropriate to seek the guidance of a specialist or more experienced nurse	In simple or common/familiar situations, is able to compare the client's data patterns with those known and to develop/explain intervention plans; has difficulty, however, with even moderately difficult data/situations that are within the expectations for students, inappropriately requires advice or assistance	Even in simple of familiar/common situations has difficulty interpreting or making sense of data; has trouble distinguishing among competing explanations and appropriate interventions, requiring assistance both in diagnosing the problem and in developing an intervention

FIGURE 5.6 — Lasater clinical judgment rubric (cont.)

Responding and Reflecting

	Exemplary	Accomplished	Developing	Beginning
Effective RESPONDING involves:				
Calm, Confident Manner	Assumes responsibility: delegates team assignments, assess the client and reassures them and their families	Generally displays leadership and confidence, and is able to control/calm most situations; may show stress in particularly difficult or complex situations	Is tentative in the leader's role; reassures clients/families in routine and relatively simple situations, but becomes stressed and disorganized easily	Except in simple and routine situations, is stressed and disorganized, lacks control, making clients and families anxious/less able to cooperate
Clear Communication	Communicates effectively; explains interventions; calms/reassures clients and families; directs and involves team members, explaining and giving directions; checks for understanding	Generally communicates well; explains carefully to clients, gives clear directions to team; could be more effective in establishing rapport	Shows some communication ability (e.g., giving directions); communication with clients/families/team members is only partly successful; displays caring but not competence	Has difficulty communicating; explanations are confusing, directions are unclear or contradictory, and clients/families are made confused/anxious, not reassured
Well-Planned Intervention/Flexibility	Interventions are tailored for the individual client; monitors client progress closely and is able to adjust treatment as indicated by the client response	Develops interventions based on relevant patient data; monitors progress regularly but does not expect to have to change treatments	Develops interventions based on the most obvious data; monitors progress, but is unable to make adjustments based on the patient response	Focuses on developing a single intervention addressing a likely solution, but it may be vague, confusing, and/or incomplete; some monitoring may occur
Being Skillful	Shows mastery of necessary nursing skills	Displays proficiency in the use of most nursing skills; could improve speed or accuracy	Is hesitant or ineffective in utilizing nursing skills	Is unable to select and/or perform the nursing skills
Effective REFLECTING involves:				
Evaluation/Self-Analysis	Independently evaluates/analyzes personal clinical performance, noting decision points, elaborating alternatives and accurately evaluating choices against alternatives	Evaluates/analyzes personal clinical performance with minimal prompting, primarily major events/decisions; key decision points are identified and alternatives are considered	Even when prompted, briefly verbalizes the most obvious evaluations; has difficulty imagining alternative choices; is self-protective in evaluating personal choices	Even prompted evaluations are brief, cursory, and not used to improve performance; justifies personal decisions/choices without evaluating them
Commitment to Improvement	Demonstrates commitment to ongoing improvement: reflects on and critically evaluates nursing experiences; accurately identifies strengths/weaknesses and develops specific plans to eliminate weaknesses	Demonstrates a desire to improve nursing performance: reflects on and evaluates experiences; identifies strengths/weaknesses; could be more systematic in evaluating weaknesses	Demonstrates awareness of the need for ongoing improvement and makes some effort to learn from experience and improve performance but tends to state the obvious, and needs external evaluation	Appears uninterested in improving performance or unable to do so; rarely reflects; is uncritical of him/herself, or overly critical (given level of development); is unable to see flaws or need for improvement

Source: Kathie Lasater. Used with permission. All rights reserved.

Self-evaluation in writing is another strategy that can be effective (Nielsen, Stragnell, and Jester 2007). For example, the facilitator may ask learners to self-rate the 11 dimensions, using the rubric, and give examples of why they rate themselves at that level (Cato, Lasater, and Peeples, in press). This, in turn, sets the stage for feedback that will help to affirm the learner and/or set goals for improvement.

Nurses are key members of the healthcare team. Based on the IOM's 2003 recommendation for nurses and other healthcare professionals to train in interprofessional teams, simulation could be an excellent pedagogical choice. The possibilities abound for interprofessional simulation. In situ settings that make sense for interprofessional development include the emergency department, the operating room, labor and delivery, and ICU, among others. The primary advantage is that healthcare professionals learn about each others' scope of practice, thereby fostering trust and communication. Getting schedules aligned and staffing covered for the period of the simulation are the primary challenges to interprofessional simulation; however, as patient safety and quality improvement issues become increasingly important, staff development specialists may appeal to executives for creative solutions to these types of issues.

There are several ways to implement simulation in the teaching setting. The variations will depend on considerations, such as infrastructure, budget, and personnel, to name a few.

Implementation on a smaller budget

Implementation of full-scale mannequin-based simulation requires a substantial initial investment. Sometimes it is difficult to help those with the fiscal responsibility for budgets to understand the value of such a financial commitment. On the other hand, the mandate for simulation may come from administrators, who then look to staff development to implement simulation without adequate resources (especially personnel). In either case, the key to gaining buy-in and managing the financial issues is a strategic plan, preferably before purchasing. Again, the intended purposes and learning outcomes must drive the plan.

Once the purposes and outcomes have been identified, other needs can be considered. Regardless of the setting in which simulation will take place, there is always the requirement for dedicated, secure storage. If there will be a center, the security of the center, including policies for who will be using the equipment, is vital. If the primary setting will be in situ, then room for storage and mobile transport mechanisms for the equipment is essential.

Given the designated outcomes, staff development specialists should consider what kind of simulation best serves the institution and plan for any equipment and supply acquisition. It may be staged over time or purchased all at once. Whatever the choice, the key is to purchase the least amount of equipment to meet the learning needs. The reverse is also true: If price is the only consideration, one could end up with equipment that does not really meet the institutional needs. After learning needs, practical considerations also must be part of the decision; for example, if in situ simulation will be the primary use, the weight and ability to transport the mannequin(s) may be an important factor that drives the ultimate purchase decision.

If the institution is part of an educational setting or a larger consortium of entities, collaboration for simulation may make cost sharing feasible. For example, a teaching hospital may collaborate with the local school of nursing to share simulation space and equipment. Community entities, such as an ambulance company or the fire department, may be willing cost-sharing partners as well.

Some states have formed alliances among entities that are using simulation as pedagogy (Oregon Simulation Alliance 2008). They are usually open to membership at relatively low cost and may offer conferences or training sessions for simulation facilitators and/or technologists, listservs for sharing ideas or new resources, and group buying arrangements. In addition to these services, online repositories for sharing scenarios and other learning activities may be a benefit. Belonging to such an organization can provide enormous support for an institution, whether its members are just starting their simulation programs or are looking for information to further develop their programs.

Training simulation team members to facilitate simulation can be a daunting task, especially for the first person designated to be a facilitator. New skill sets are required in order to promote learning through simulation (Jeffries 2008). Training opportunities may range from observing simulation at a nearby academic or service institution, availing oneself of online course modules, attending the training offered by the mannequin vendors, taking academic courses that integrate simulation into a staff development program to hiring a training consultant. The best simulation training comes from having the most opportunity for hands-on experiences. For additional personnel, it may be important to consider the return on investment (ROI); that is, with more experience, the less dependence on outside resources is necessary.

Ultimately, organizations need a way to evaluate their ROI, preferably before purchase and certainly after. This is why the pre-determination of intended learner outcomes is so crucial. As high-fidelity simulators become more sophisticated in their technology and realism, the feature options become more numerous and confusing. Vendors are only too happy to share the range of attractive features that are available. Knowing the learning outcomes before buying can assist in determining which features are necessities, which would be nice to have, and which are completely unnecessary for the individual program. Smart planning to identify priorities, taking time to review and compare the features between mannequins, and conferring with consultants and other experts who are not stakeholders are all strategies that will ensure the highest ROI.

Once again, the intended learning outcomes drive the evaluation strategies. For example, if advancing patient safety or reducing error is the primary outcome, one might evaluate the effectiveness of using simulation for this purpose by observing the rates of patient accidents or incident reports of errors to see whether changes have occurred. Increasing numbers of new grads have been exposed to simulation during their academic experiences; they might expect to continue learning in this manner. Using simulation as a learning tool may increase the satisfaction among nursing staff, which may, in turn, increase staff retention, an important potential ROI.

Evaluating your options

As we've outlined in this chapter, there are many simulation options to consider and from which to choose. You want the best for your institution, both operationally as well as to benefit the nursing and other healthcare staff members. Given accreditation requirements for institutional staff development and your organization's ongoing focus on patient safety, the decisions about using different simulation strategies must be win-win for the institution as well as the staff it employs and supports.

Deciding on the right technology

Throughout the chapter, we discussed the many factors that must be considered when choosing the best simulation strategies for your institution; these include the intended learning outcomes, the available space in your facility, scheduling and time constraints, available personnel for facilitation, and, of course, budget.

One way to begin to evaluate your choice(s) is to gather information about all of these factors to see what is possible. Phasing in mannequin-based simulation over a period of time may well be part of the plan (e.g., beginning with one mannequin suitable for the greatest training need and using it in situ). Knowing the intended learning outcomes is a critical beginning place for considering any kind of teaching strategy.

Justifying your resources

More often than not, the catalyst for justifying simulation is the staff development specialist. Justification requires a thorough assessment of each of the factors above and pulling together a plan to show how simulation, in whatever form, can foster those learning outcomes and give the desired ROI. For example, if simulation-based training results in fewer errors and better team-work, the institution will benefit. Often, the strategic plan for the institution can offer assistance for dovetailing needs; in other words, if your plan can support other mandates, such as impor-tant safety initiatives, you are more likely to be able to justify beginning a simulation program.

Similarly, if one of your institution's strategies is to strengthen relationships with a local academic institution, a plan for beginning a shared simulation program may be a key accomplishment. Convene a group of all the stakeholders, including your foundation or development executive, to creatively determine how to present the plan to administration as well as carry it out.

Obtaining administrative buy-in

If you can show administration how simulation, though expensive to begin (in the case of mannequin-based), can be cost-effective over a period of time in retaining nursing staff or reducing the number of other required training to meet the mandates of the strategic plan, you will be likely to gain its support and buy-in.

For ongoing administrative support, it is essential to collect information and data to sustain your simulation program. This can be in the form of course evaluations to demonstrate achieve-ment of your learning outcomes or also in the larger sense of program data reporting. Keeping track of data, such as the numbers and types of simulation strategies, hours spent, and personnel needed, are essential in painting that larger picture to the executives who do not witness the daily operations of a facility. Additionally, consider inviting stakeholders to see how simulation works. The old adage of a picture being worth a thousand words applies here. Disseminating participant stories by sharing testimonials may also be a useful strategy.

Obtaining staff buy-in

Nursing and other healthcare staff members may also need to be won over. Nurses, in particular, are in short supply and are directly tied to patient care, so simulation may seem like one more demand. Taking the opportunity to carefully plan for the introduction of simulation will pay off because you want your first healthcare staff to have positive experiences. Find out what is most important to them as part of your overall plan. Also, talk with staff members one-on-one, providing information about simulation research, utilization, and best evidence specific to their concerns. Consider these additional strategies to create buy-in for simulation at both administrative and staff levels:

- Partner and collaborate with others through professional organizations (e.g., the National League for Nursing)

- Send simulation facilitators to participate or present at local and national conferences

- Develop champions by sending them to national meetings, training, and workshops

- Communicate results and make simulation visible through pictures, presentations, and articles

New Technology in Nursing Staff Development

References

Accreditation Council for Graduate Medical Education. (2008). Resident duty hours-standards. Retrieved August 2, 2008 from *http://www.acgme.org/acWebsite/navPages/nav_residents.asp.*

Alinier, G. (2008). *Professional stage craft: How to create simulated clinical environments out of smoke and mirrors.* In Kyle, R., and Murray, W. (Eds.). *Clinical simulation operations, engineering and management.* Burlington, MA: Elsevier. 701–712.

American Nurses Credentialing Center. (2008). Nurse magnet program. Retrieved July 29, 2008, from *www.nursecredentialing.org.*

Benner, P. (1984). From novice to expert: *Excellence and power in clinical nursing practice.* San Francisco: Addison-Wesley.

Benner, P., Chesla, C., and Tanner, C. (1996). *Expertise in nursing: Caring, clinical judgment, and ethics.* New York: Springer Publishing Company.

Billings, D. and Halstead, J. (1998). *Teaching in nursing: A guide for faculty.* St. Louis: Saunders.

Boud, D., Keogh, R., and Walker, D. (1985). *Reflection: Turning experience into learning.* London: Kogan Page.

Cato, M., Lasater, K., and Peeples, A. (in press). "Student nurses' self-assessment of their simulation experiences." *Nursing Education Perspectives.*

Christensen, U. (2006). "Microsimulation (PC Simulation) in emergency health care learning and assessment." *International TraumaCare* 16(1): 12–18.

Craft, M. (2005). "Reflective writing and nursing education." *Journal of Nursing Education* 44(2): 53–57.

Cross, K. (1998). "Why learning communities? Why now?" *About Campus* 3(3): 4–11.

del Bueno, D. (2005). "A crisis in critical thinking." *Nursing Education Perspectives* 26(5): 278–282.

Dewey, J. (1933). *How we think: A restatement of the relation of reflective thinking to the educative process.* Chicago: Henry Regnery.

Driggers, B. (2008, July 14). Simulation history and trends. Presented at Oregon Health & Science University School of Nursing Intensive, Teaching Clinical Judgment through Simulation: An Intensive Workshop for Nurse Educators. Portland, OR.

Gomez, G., and Gomez, E. (1987). "Learning of psychomotor skills: Laboratory versus patient care setting." *Journal of Nursing Education* 26(1): 20–24.

Harden, R., and Stamper, N. (1999). "What is a spiral curriculum?" *Medical Teacher* 21(2): 141–143.

Hertel, J., and Millis, B. (2002). Using simulations to promote learning in higher education: An introduction. Sterling, VA: Stylus Publishing.

Hovanscek, M. (2007). *Using simulation in nursing education.* In P. Jeffries (Ed.), *Simulation in nursing education: From conceptualization to evaluation.* New York: National League for Nursing. 1–9.

Institute of Medicine. (1999). To err is human: Building a safer health system. Committee on Quality of Health Care in America.

Institute of Medicine. (2003). Health professions education: A bridge to quality. Retrieved October 11, 2003, from *www.iom.edu/report*.

Jeffries, P. (2008). "Getting in S.T.E.P. with simulations: Simulations take educator preparation." *Nursing Education Perspectives* 29(2): 70–73.

Jeffries, P., and Rogers, K. (2007). *Theoretical framework for simulation design*. In P. Jeffries (Ed.), *Simulation in nursing education: From conceptualization to evaluation* (pp. 21–33). New York: National League for Nursing.

Jenkins, L., Shaivone, K., Budd, N., Waltz, C., and Griffith, K. (2006). "Educational innovations: Use of genitorurinary teaching associates (GUTAs) to teach nurse practitioner students: is self-efficacy theory a useful framework?" *Journal of Nursing Education* 45(1): 35–37.

Johnson and Johnson on Health Care Systems, Inc. (2003). Discover nursing. Retrieved June 9, 2003, from *http://www.discovernursing.com/market.asp*.

Kolb, D. (1984). *Experiential learning: Experience as the source of learning and development*. Englewood Cliffs, NJ: Prentice-Hall.

Lasater, K. (2007a). "High fidelity simulation and the development of clinical judgment: Student experiences." *Journal of Nursing Education* 46: 269–276.

Lasater, K. (2007b). "Clinical judgment development: Using simulation to create an assessment rubric." *Journal of Nursing Education* 46: 496–503.

Lasater, K., and Nielsen, A. (in press). "Reflective journaling for clinical judgment development and evaluation." *Journal of Nursing Education*.

Lederman, J. (1992). "Debriefing: Toward a systematic assessment of theory and practice." *Simulation & Gaming* 23: 145–160.

Murphy, J. (2004). "Using focused reflection and articulation to promote clinical reasoning: An evidence-based teaching strategy." *Nursing Education Perspectives* 25(5): 226–231.

Nielsen, A., Stragnell, S., and Jester, P. (2007). "Guide for reflection using the clinical judgment model." *Journal of Nursing Education* 46(11): 513–516.

Oregon Simulation Alliance. (2008). Oregon Simulation Alliance. Retrieved July 29, 2008, from *www.oregonsimulation.com*.

Porter-O'Grady, T. (2001). "Profound change: 21st century nursing." *Nursing Outlook* 49(4):182–186.

Rall, M., Stricker, E., Reddersen, S., Zieger, J., and Dieckmann, P. (2008). *"In situ" simulation crisis resource management training*. In Kyle, R., and Murray, W. (Eds.). *Clinical simulation operations, engineering and management*. Burlington, MA: Elsevier. 565–581.

Rentschler, D., Eaton, J., Cappiello, J., McNally, S., and McWilliam, P. (2007). "Evaluation of undergraduate students using objective structured clinical evaluation." *Journal of Nursing Education* 46(3): 135–139.

Salas, E., Wilson, K., Burke, C., and Priest. H. (2005). "Using simulation-based training to improve patient safety: What does it take?" *Journal on Quality and Patient Safety* 31(7): 363–371.

Seropian, M., Brown, K., Gavilanes, J., and Driggers, B. (2004). "Simulation: Not just a manikin." *Journal of Nursing Education*, 43, 164–169.

Seropian, M., Dillman, D., Lasater, K., and Gavilanes, J. (2007). "Mannequin-based simulation to reinforce pharmacology concepts: Where theory meets practice." *Simulation in Healthcare* 2(4): 218–233.

Spunt, D. (2007). *Setting up a simulation laboratory.* In P. Jeffries (Ed.). *Simulation in nursing education: From conceptualization to evaluation.* New York: National League for Nursing. 105–122.

Tanner, C. (2005). "What have we learned about critical thinking in nursing?" *Journal of Nursing Education* 44: 47–48.

Tanner, C. (2006). "Thinking like a nurse: A research-based model of clinical judgment." *Journal of Nursing Education* 45: 204–211.

The Joint Commission. (2008). *The Joint Commission Comprehensive Accreditation Manual for Hospitals.* Standards. Oakbrook Terrace, IL: Joint Commission Resources, Inc.

Additional resources

Books

Hertel, J., and Millis, B. (2002). *Using simulations to promote learning in higher education: An introduction*. Sterling, VA: Stylus Publishing.

Jeffries, P. (Ed.). (2007). *Simulation in nursing education: From conceptualization to evaluation*. New York: National League for Nursing.

Kyle, R., and Murray, W. (Eds.). (2008). *Clinical simulation operations, engineering and management*. Burlington, MA: Elsevier.

Simulation organizations

International Nursing Association for Clinical Simulation and Learning. Retrieved July 31, 2008, from *www.inacsl.org*.

Society for Simulation in Healthcare. Retrieved July 31, 2008, from *www.ssih.org*.

Online course modules

Simulation Innovation Resource Center. Retrieved July 29, 2008, from *www.nln.org/sirc*.

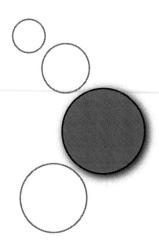

Nursing education instructional guide

Target audience

- Staff educators

- Directors of education

- Staff development specialists

- Organizational development specialists

- Directors of nursing

- Vice Presidents of nursing

- Chief nursing officers

Statement of need

This book explains how to use different types of new technology and how to choose the right nontraditional methods for an organization. Techniques presented in this book will help educators master these cutting-edge options and stretch their training dollars by justifying certain techniques. The accompanying CD-ROM includes all the customizable tools and forms found in the book.

Educational objectives

Upon completion of this activity, participants should be able to:

- Identify advantages of teaching with audio/visual (A/V) technologies

- List roadblocks that may hinder the use of A/V media

- Describe the technological necessities for developing Webcasts

- Determine benefits of Web conferencing

- List four of the most common types of Web-based communication

- Discuss copyright considerations in relation to Web-based training

- Identify methods for overcoming barriers in blended learning

- Discuss the role of the multigenerational classroom in blended learning

- List the benefits of using simulation as a staff training tool

Faculty

Diane Billings, EdD, RN, FAAN—Diane Billings is chancellors' professor emeritus of nursing at Indiana University School of Nursing in Indianapolis, IN. She is the reviewer of this publication.

Dorothea Devanna, MS, ACNS-BC—Dorothea Devanna is a medical-surgical clinical nurse specialist at Mount Auburn Hospital in Cambridge, MA. She is an author for this publication.

Jesika Gavilanes, MA—Jesika Gavilanes is the operations manager of the Oregon Health and Science University (OHSU) simulation and clinical learning center. She is an author for this publication.

Cynthia Hollingsworth, MS, BS, AAS—Cynthia Hollingsworth is the coordinator of instructional design and an adjunct assistant faculty at the Indiana University School of Nursing in Indianapolis, IN. She is an author for this publication.

Kathie Lasater, EdD, RN—Kathie Lasater is an assistant professor at the Oregon Health and Science University (OHSU) School of Nursing in Portland. She is an author for this publication.

Nursing continuing education:

This educational activity for three contact hours is provided by HCPro, Inc.

HCPro is accredited as a provider of continuing nursing education by the American Nurses Credentialing Center's (ANCC) Commission on Accreditation.

Disclosure statements

HCPro Inc. has confirmed that none of the faculty/presenters or contributors have any relevant financial relationships to disclose related to the content of this educational activity.

Instructions

In order to be eligible to receive your nursing contact hour(s) for this activity, you are required to do the following:

1. Read the book

2. Complete the exam

3. Complete the evaluation

4. Provide your contact information in the space provided on the exam and evaluation

5. Submit the exam and evaluation to HCPro.

Please provide all of the information requested above and mail or fax your completed exam, program evaluation, and contact information to:

HCPro, Inc.
ATTN: Continuing Education Department
200 Hoods Lane
Marblehead, MA 01945
Tel: 877/727-1728
Fax: 781/639-2982

Nursing education exam

_____

Name

_____

Title

_____

Facility name

_____

Address 1

_____

Address 2

_____

City   State

_____

ZIP

_____

Phone number   Fax number

_____

E-mail

_____

Nursing license number

(ANCC requires a unique identifier for each learner.)

1.   One advantage of commercial videos is that they are:

    a.   portable   c.   amateur

    b.   complicated   d.   ageless

2.   The term "podcast" was first attributed to Ben Hammersley in 2004 by combining what two terms?

    a.   "Portable" and "casting"   c.   "Tripod" and "newscast"

    b.   "iPod" and "broadcast"   d   "Pod" and "castaway"

3. **Which of the following is a potential roadblock in using A/V media?**

    a. Institutions will usually find the technology difficult to implement

    b. Publishers may be reluctant to grant permission for commercially created media

    c. The technologies are not often transportable

    d. Professional actors are always necessary for videos

4. **What is a significant drawback in the use of DVDs as teaching tools?**

    a. They are not portable

    b. The content does not easily load

    c. Poor visual clarity

    d. The content may be dated

5. **Which of the following is NOT an essential component you'd need to implement Web conferencing?**

    a. Screen sharing

    b. Chat

    c. Whiteboard

    d. Telephone

6. **The terms "Web conferencing" and _____ are often used synonymously as their capabilities are becoming more and more similar.**

    a. "online conferencing"

    b. "video conferencing"

    c. "virtual conferencing"

    d. "DVD conferencing"

7. **Web conferencing can be an ideal solution if you have:**

    a. an out-of-town interviewee

    b. a writing-for-publication obligation

    c. new budgeting strategies

    d. limited computer configuration

8. **The polling function of a Web conference allows participants to ask ____ questions.**

    a. on-the-fly

    b. delayed

    c. unrelated

    d. limited

9. **All of the following are a common type of Web-based communication EXCEPT:**

   a. discussion forums

   b. announcements

   c. mail

   d. clipboards

10. **_____ is a real-time, synchronous mode of communication.**

    a. Voice mail

    b. Chat

    c. E-mail

    d. Billing

11. **Everything that is created and is stored in a _____ is copyrighted by the author/ creator/developer.**

    a. open medium

    b. fixed process

    c. fixed medium

    d. open process

12. **Julie recently published an article in a nursing journal. She wishes to republish some of the material from the article. Who most likely owns the copyright to this material?**

    a. Julie

    b. The journal

    c. Julie's facility

    d. No one owns the copyright

13. **Which of the following is an effective method for training an auditory learner?**

    a. Lectures

    b. Printouts

    c. Simulation

    d. Posters

14. **A visual impairment in a classroom is an example of what kind of barrier to blended learning?**

    a. Physical

    b. Attitude

    c. Cognitive

    d. Sensory

15. **Members of which generational group often spend significant time surfing the Internet?**

    a. Veterans

    b. Generation X

    c. Generation Y

    d. Baby boomers

16. **The classroom environment for Veterans often consisted of the following EXCEPT:**

    a. reading materials   c. lectures

    b. written tests   d. computers

17. **Which generation was often viewed as a group of "overachievers?"**

    a. Baby boomers   c. Generation X

    b. Veterans   d. Generation Y

18. **High-tech simulation mannequins often have patient characteristics, EXCEPT for:**

    a. a pulse   c. realistic anatomy

    b. breathing sounds   d. thought capability

19. **Beyond the mannequin or body part task trainer, simulation fidelity can be enhanced by attending to the details within the environment. This is sometimes referred to as _____ fidelity.**

    a. physical   c. psychological

    b. emotional   d. spiritual

20. **Role-play may be the most desired form of simulation when dealing with what type of patient?**

    a. Collaborative   c. Unemotional

    b. Combative   d. Cheerful

Nursing education evaluation

Name

Title

Facility name

Address 1

Address 2

City   State   ZIP

Phone number   Fax number

E-mail

Nursing license number

(ANCC requires a unique identifier for each learner)

1.   This activity met the following learning objectives:

a.   Identify advantages of teaching with A/V technologies

Strongly disagree   1   2   3   4   5   Strongly agree

b.   List roadblocks that may hinder the use of A/V media

Strongly disagree   1   2   3   4   5   Strongly agree

c.   Describe the technological necessities for developing Webcasts

Strongly disagree   1   2   3   4   5   Strongly agree

                       New Technology in Nursing Staff Development

d. Determine benefits of Web conferencing

Strongly disagree   1   2   3   4   5   Strongly agree

e. List four of the most common types of Web-based communication

Strongly disagree   1   2   3   4   5   Strongly agree

f. Discuss copyright considerations in relation to Web-based training

Strongly disagree   1   2   3   4   5   Strongly agree

g. Identify methods for overcoming barriers in blended learning

Strongly disagree   1   2   3   4   5   Strongly agree

h. Discuss the role of the multigenerational classroom in blended learning

Strongly disagree   1   2   3   4   5   Strongly agree

i. List the benefits of using simulation as a staff training tool

Strongly disagree   1   2   3   4   5   Strongly agree

2. Objectives were related to the overall purpose/goal of the activity.

Strongly disagree   1   2   3   4   5   Strongly agree

3. This activity was related to my nursing activity needs.

Strongly disagree   1   2   3   4   5   Strongly agree

4. The exam for the activity was an accurate test of the knowledge gained.

Strongly disagree   1   2   3   4   5   Strongly agree

5. The activity avoided commercial bias or influence.

Strongly disagree   1   2   3   4   5   Strongly agree

6. **This activity met my expectations.**

    Strongly disagree   1   2   3   4   5   Strongly agree

7. **Will this learning activity enhance your professional nursing practice?**

    Yes   No

8. **This educational method was an appropriate delivery tool for the nursing/clinical audience.**

    Strongly disagree   1   2   3   4   5   Strongly agree

9. **How committed are you to making the behavioral changes suggested in this activity?**

    a. Very committed

    b. Somewhat committed

    c. Not committed

10. **Please provide us with your degree.**

    a. ADN

    b. BSN

    c. MSN

    d. Other, please state

11. **Please provide us with your credentials.**

    a. LVN

    b. LPN

    c. RN

    d. NP

    e. Other, please state

12. **Providing nursing contact hours for this product influenced my decision to buy it.**

    Strongly disagree   1   2   3   4   5   Strongly agree

13. **I found the process to obtain my continuing education (CE) credits for this activity easy to complete.**

        Strongly disagree   1   2   3   4   5   Strongly agree

14. **If you did not find the process easy to complete, which of the following areas did you find the most difficult?**

        a.   Understanding the content of the activity

        b.   Understanding the instructions

        c.   Completing the exam

        d.   Completing the evaluation

        e.   Other, please state:

15. **How much time did it take for you to complete this activity (this includes reading the book and completing the exam and the evaluation)?** _____

16. **If you have any comments on this activity, process, or selection of topics for nursing CE, please note them below.**

    _____

    _____

    _____

    _____

17. **Would you be interested in participating as a pilot tester for the development of future HCPro nursing education activities?**

        Yes   No

Thank you for completing this evaluation of our nursing CE activity!